Blood Collection in Healthcare

Marjorie Schaub Di Lorenzo, MT(ASCP)SH

Adjunct Medical Technology Instructor
Division of Medical Technology
School of Allied Health Professions
University of Nebraska Medical Center
Omaha, Nebraska

Phlebotomy Program Coordinator
Continuing Education
Nebraska Methodist College
Omaha, Nebraska

Susan King Strasinger, DA, MT(ASCP)

Visiting Assistant Professor
The University of West Florida
Pensacola, Florida

ILLUSTRATIONS BY:

Sherman Bonomelli, MS
Medical Technology Program
The University of West Florida
Pensacola, Florida

PHOTOGRAPHY BY:

Frankie Harris-Lyne, MLT(ASCP), CLS(NCA)
Instructor/Clinical Coordinator
MLT and Phlebotomy Programs
Northern Virginia Community College
Annandale, Virginia

F. A. Davis Company • Philadelphia

F. A. Davis Company
1915 Arch Street
Philadelphia, PA 19103
www.fadavis.com

Printed in the United States of America

Last digit indicates print number: 10 9 8 7 6 5 4 3 2

Acquisitions Editor: Christa Fratantoro
Developmental Editor: Christa Fratantoro
Production Editor: Nwakaego Fletcher-Perry
Cover Designer: Louis Forgione

As new scientific information becomes available through basic and clinical research, recommended treatments and drug therapies undergo changes. The author(s) and publisher have done everything possible to make this book accurate, up to date, and in accord with accepted standards at the time of publication. The author(s), editors, and publisher are not responsible for errors or omissions or for consequences from application of the book, and make no warranty, expressed or implied, in regard to the contents of the book. Any practice described in this book should be applied by the reader in accordance with professional standards of care used in regard to the unique circumstances that may apply in each situation. The reader is advised always to check product information (package inserts) for changes and new information regarding dose and contraindications before administering any drug. Caution is especially urged when using new or infrequently ordered drugs.

Library of Congress Cataloging-in-Publication Data

Di Lorenzo, Marjorie Schaub, 1953-

Blood collection in healthcare / Marjorie Schaub Di Lorenzo, Susan King Strasinger.

    p. cm.
    Includes bibliographical references and index.
    ISBN 0-8036-0848-9 (pbk.)
    1. Blood-Collection and preservation. 2. Phlebotomy.   I.
Strasinger, Susan King.   II. Title
RB45. 15 .D525 2001
616.07′561—dc21
     2001028564

To my husband, Scott,
and my children, Michael, Christopher, and Lauren

MSD

To Harry,
my Editor-in-Chief

SKS

Preface

This short course textbook is designed to provide practicing health-care personnel with concise information on the proper techniques to collect quality blood specimens with minimal patient discomfort. The purpose of the book, *Blood Collection in Healthcare,* is primarily for the cross training and continuing education of health-care professionals currently performing phlebotomy work or those who anticipate performing phlebotomy procedures in the future. Today's concept of developing health-care teams to help streamline patient care has evolved to encompass the cross training of nurses, respiratory therapists, radiology technologists, medical assistants, clinical nursing assistants, and medical technologists. Phlebotomy has become a major part of this cross training.

Topics emphasized in the text include: the types of blood required for specific lab tests, the purpose of these tests, vein selection and alternate sites, types of collection tubes and the purpose of anticoagulants, order of draw, test-specific handling, complications and remedies, and storage and transportation conditions. Information common to all health-care curriculums, such as safety precautions, anatomy and physiology, quality assurance, and patient-caregiver interactions, is covered only in the context of their relationship to the collection of blood specimens.

This current comprehensive text provides a cost-effective, compact learning tool for phlebotomy short courses. Highlighted features of this text include learning objectives; blood collection equipment, including the newest safety devices; technical procedures for venipuncture and dermal puncture; special collection procedures, including access to central venous catheters; specimen handling, storage, and transport procedures; and technical tips to avoid complications such as hematomas and hemolysis. Methods to increase the quality of blood specimens, correlation of laboratory tests and clinical disorders, safety precautions, and quality assurance procedures required by laboratory regulatory agencies as they relate to phlebotomy are emphasized. Numerous illustrations, photographs, diagrams, charts, and tables visually enhance the comprehension of complex information and technical procedures. Practical situation problem-solving exercises, performance evaluation checklists for technical procedures, and a self-assessment examination reinforce information. All procedures are written to comply with the standards set forth by the Occupational Safety and Health Administration, the Joint Commission on Accreditation of Healthcare Organizations, and the National Committee for Clinical Laboratory Standards.

This text provides a quick reference for blood collection skills. Appendices list reference material such as frequently ordered laboratory tests with the required types of anticoagulants and volume of blood required and IV access flush protocols. A summary of laboratory tests, their function, and their clinical correlation is included. Answer keys for the situation problem-solving and self-assessment sections are also available. A complete color tube guide lists all the different types of collection tubes, the additives, number of inversions required, and laboratory uses of the tubes. Chapter outlines are included to facilitate instruction. A Power Point presentation provides instructors with an additional instructional tool.

We specifically designed this text to meet the need of nurses and other health-care professionals who want and need to add a new phlebotomy competency or to reinforce past learned skills. It can be used to promote learning in academic settings, hospital training sessions, or continuing education courses.

ADDITIONAL REFERENCES

National Committee for Clinical Laboratory Standards. Procedure for the Collection of Diagnostic Blood Specimens by Venipuncture, ed. 4. Approved Standard, H3-A4, NCCLS, Villanova, PA, 1998

National Committee for Clinical Laboratory Standards. Procedure for the Handling and Processing of Blood Specimens, Approved Guideline, H18-A2, NCCLS, Villanova, PA, 1999.

National Committee for Clinical Laboratory Standards. Procedure for the Collection of Diagnostic Blood Specimens by Skin Puncture, ed. 4. H4-A4, NCCLS, Villanova, PA, 1999.

Strasinger, SK and Di Lorenzo, MS. Phlebotomy Workbook for the Multiskilled Healthcare Professional. FA Davis, Philadelphia, 1996.

ADDITIONAL TEACHING AIDS

VIDEOTAPES

Quality Venipuncture: The Key to Accurate Results, H3-A4-V
Quality Microcollection, H4-A3-V
Available from NCCLS
(1-877-447-1888)

Blood Collection: Modern Blood Collection Techniques for Nurses
Becton Dickinson Education Center
1 Becton Drive
Franklin Lakes, NJ 07417
1-800-255-6334

Blood Collection: Microcollection Techniques
Becton Dickinson Education Center
1 Becton Drive
Franklin Lakes, NJ 07417
1-800-255-6334

Blood Collection: The Difficult Draw
Becton Dickinson Education Center
1 Becton Drive
Franklin Lakes, NJ 07417
1-800-255-6334

Blood Collection: Troubleshooting and Helpful Hints
Becton Dickinson Education Center
1 Becton Drive
Franklin Lakes, NJ 07417
1-800-255-6334

Blood Collection: Transportation & Helpful Hints
Becton Dickinson Education Center
1 Becton Drive
Franklin Lakes, NJ 07417
1-800-255-6334

Blood Collection: Product Information
Becton Dickinson Education Center
1 Becton Drive
Franklin Lakes, NJ 07417
1-800-255-6334

CD-ROM

Phlebotomy Tutor
Educational Software, Lippincott
University of Washington
Department of Laboratory Medicine

Acknowledgements

We wish to thank Diane Wolff, MT (ASCP), the phlebotomy team leader, and Patty Janousek, BSN, CRNI, the IV Team Leader at Methodist Hospital, Omaha, Nebraska for their expertise and valuable charts used in the appendices; and Joey Caraway, MT (ASCP) and Troy Lewis, MT (ASCP) at Sacred Heart Hospital, Pensacola, Florida for their encouragement and providing access to NCCLS publications. We are particularly grateful to Sherman Bonomelli from the University of West Florida, Pensacola, Florida for preparing the Power Point presentation that accompanies this text.

Reviewers

Terry Kotrla, MT(ASCP)BB
Associate Professor
MLT and Phlebotomy Programs
Austin Community College
Austin, Texas

Frankie Harris-Lyne, MLT(ASCP), CLS(NCA)
Instructor/Clinical Coordinator
MLT and Phlebotomy Programs
Northern Virginia Community College
Annandale, Virginia

Gary B. Pickett, MS, MT(ASCP)
Professor & Director
Medical Laboratory Technology & Phlebotomy Programs
West Virginia Northern Community College
Wheeling, West Virginia

James E. Daly, BS, MEd, MT(ASCP)
Associate Professor/Program Director
CLS Tech/Phlebotomy Programs
Lorain County Community College
Elyria, Ohio

Jay W. Wilborn, MEd, CLS
MLT-AD Program Director
Garland County Community College
Hot Springs, Arkansas

John H. Clouse, MSR, R.T.(R)
Associate Professor of Radiology
Owensboro Community College
Owensboro, Kentucky

Larry Dean Jobe, A.S., R.T.(R)
Instructor
Hendrick Medical Center
School of Radiography
Abilene, Texas

Debra K. Kasel, M.Ed., RRT
Assistant Professor of Respiratory Care
Northern Kentucky University
Highland Heights, Kentucky

Contents

U·N·I·T 1

Introduction to Blood Collection

Learning Objectives

Upon completion of this unit, the reader will be able to:

☐ Recognize the importance of correct blood collection techniques in total patient care.

☐ Discuss safety precautions as related to blood collection.

☐ List the factors that influence the integrity of a blood specimen.

☐ Differentiate between whole blood, plasma, and serum.

☐ Explain the action of anticoagulants to prevent blood coagulation.

☐ Describe the appearance of a hemolyzed, icteric, and lipemic specimen.

☐ Differentiate between arterial, venous, and capillary blood.

☐ State the purpose of quality assurance in blood collection.

INTRODUCTION

The redesigning of the health-care system to obtain more efficient and cost-effective patient care has resulted in many changes in personnel responsibilities. One of the major changes has been the shifting of blood specimen collection from phlebotomists based in the clinical laboratory to nursing service personnel and other allied health professionals.

Consequently, many health-care personnel are now required to become proficient in a skill for which they have had little or no previous exposure. Like any other skill, collection of quality blood specimens begins by obtaining the didactic knowledge associated with the procedure. This is followed by performance of the skill with assistance and supervision. Adhering to proper technique and continued practice then becomes the key to acquiring proficiency.

IMPORTANCE OF CORRECT SPECIMEN COLLECTION AND HANDLING

Laboratory testing of blood specimens is vital to the diagnosis, treatment, and monitoring of a patient's condition. The quality of a test result is only as good as the quality of the specimen analyzed. Therefore, reports from a suboptimal specimen can result in treatment that can be potentially harmful to the patient.

Laboratories are charged with the responsibility for specimen integrity by the Clinical Laboratory Improvement Amendments (CLIA, 1988). Guidelines for specimen collection are published by the laboratory and should be available in all areas where patient samples are collected. Personnel collecting specimens should become familiar with these guidelines and refer to them or call the laboratory whenever they are unsure of a procedure.

Although the primary concern of personnel collecting blood specimens is understandably to obtain the specimen, failure to adhere to the collection procedure can compromise the integrity of a successfully collected specimen. Responsibilities of the blood collector also include:

- Correct patient identification
- Patient preparation
- Timing of collections
- Collection techniques
- Specimen labeling
- Specimen transportation to the laboratory

It is these ancillary factors that most frequently affect specimen integrity, resulting in specimen rejection by the laboratory. Therefore, emphasis in this course is placed on both technical and nontechnical factors that must be included in quality blood specimen collection.

SAFETY PRECAUTIONS

In addition to the safety precautions specifically associated with blood collection, which are covered in this text, personnel must observe all standard precautions required in patient care. This includes:

- Wearing appropriate personnel protective equipment (PPE)
- Observation of isolation practices
- Handwashing
- Disposal of contaminated materials in designated biohazard containers
- Decontamination of surfaces using an approved disinfectant, such as sodium hypochlorite (diluted 1:10), on a daily basis

Blood collection poses a serious risk for exposure to blood-borne pathogens, such as human immunodeficiency virus (HIV), hepatitis B, and hepatitis C. Standard precautions must be strictly observed. The Occupational Safety and Health Administration (OSHA) mandates that gloves be worn at all times when collecting blood specimens. Gloves must be changed and hands washed between patients. Gowns or lab coats are recommended apparel.

Most blood-borne pathogen exposures associated with blood collection occur as a result of accidental puncture with a contaminated needle or lancet. A major significant exposure occurs when a deep puncture is caused by a needle that has been used to collect blood. Therefore, strict adherence to all safety precautions is essential.

Never recap needles and always discard them in puncture-resistant containers located close to the patient. A variety of safety devices for needle disposal and also a variety of protective needle sheaths are available (see Unit 2, Venipuncture Equipment). It is extremely important that personnel become totally familiar with the use of these safety devices. Many accidental punctures occur because personnel do not know how to properly use the available safety devices.

Blood collected using a syringe must be transferred to the appropriate evacuated tubes. This presents an additional safety risk, because the recommended transfer procedure is to puncture the rubber stopper of the evacuated tube with the syringe needle and allow the blood to flow into the tube. Removal of the rubber stopper, adding the blood from the syringe, and restoppering the tube is not recommended, because aerosols are produced and tubes are not as tightly stoppered for transport. As will be demonstrated in Unit 2, the evacuated tube must be placed in a rack and not held in the hand during this procedure. A well-stocked blood collection tray contains racks for tubes, needle disposal units, and additional supplies (see Unit 2). Therefore, a blood collection tray should be placed within close proximity to the patient whenever blood is being collected.

Personnel working in off-site facilities or physicians' offices may be required to perform initial specimen processing, such as centrifugation and separation of serum or plasma from blood cells. Centrifugation of uncapped tubes produces potentially harmful aerosols. Tubes must be carefully balanced in the centrifuge to prevent breakage, and the centrifuge lid must remain closed during operation to protect workers from exposure to blood and glass should a breakage occur. To prevent aerosol exposure when removing stoppers from evacuated tubes, first cover the stopper with gauze and then twist rather than "pop" off. Aerosols are also produced when specimens are poured rather than pipetted during transfer between tubes.

Blood collection is safely performed only when personnel adhere to all recommended precautions.

Technical Tip

Needles used for blood collection have a greater potential for transmitting blood-borne pathogens than do needles used for other purposes. Report *all* needlesticks.

TYPES OF SPECIMENS

The laboratory refers to blood specimens primarily in terms of whole blood, plasma, and serum. A whole blood specimen contains erythrocytes, leukocytes, and platelets suspended in plasma and essentially represents blood as it circulates through the body. Tests related to blood cells, such as the complete blood count (CBC) and blood typing, are performed on whole blood.

The majority of laboratory tests are performed on the liquid portion of blood (plasma or serum), which contains substances such as proteins, enzymes, organic and inorganic chemicals, and antibodies. Plasma is the liquid portion of blood that has not clotted; serum is the liquid portion remaining after clotting has occurred. Plasma is often defined as the liquid portion of blood that contains fibrinogen and other clotting factors, and serum as the liquid portion that does not contain fibrinogen and other clotting factors. Both serum and plasma are obtained by centrifugation of clotted and unclotted specimens, which separates the cellular elements from the liquid portion (Figure 1–1).

The presence or absence of anticoagulants in the tubes into which blood specimens are placed determines the type of specimen available for testing. Whole

Figure 1-1

Differences between plasma and serum

(From Strasinger, SK, and Di Lorenzo, MA: Phlebotomy Workbook for the Multi-skilled Healthcare Professional. FA Davis, Philadelphia, 1996, Figure 4-2, p. 40, with permission.)

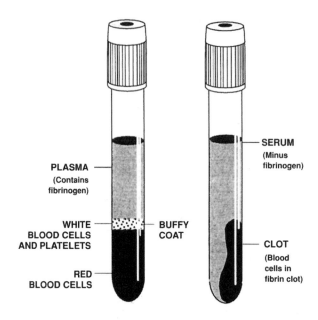

blood and plasma require an anticoagulant to prevent clot formation. Serum is obtained from tubes that do not contain anticoagulant.

Collection tubes contain a variety of anticoagulants, the chemical content of which must be considered in conjunction with the laboratory test requested. As shown in Figure 1–2, anticoagulants prevent coagulation by two different mechanisms. The anticoagulants dipotassium (K_2) and tripotassium (K_3) ethylenediaminetetraacetic acid (EDTA), sodium citrate, and potassium and ammonium oxalate bind calcium, which is required by the coagulation cascade. Heparin in the form of sodium, ammonium, or lithium heparin inhibits the formation of thrombin, which is required to convert fibrinogen into a fibrin clot.

With the obvious exception of coagulation tests, many laboratory tests can be performed on either serum or plasma. However, the anticoagulant composition and method of action must be considered when tests are to be run on plasma. For example, an EDTA tube cannot be used when a plasma calcium level is requested, because the plasma calcium will be bound to the EDTA, resulting in falsely decreased values. Normal values of some analytes also differ between serum and plasma. Laboratory protocols for specimen collection specify the type of tube to be used. These protocols have been designed to ensure that the most representative test results are obtained, and they should be followed.

Normal serum and plasma appear clear and pale yellow. Variations in the normal appearance can indicate that certain test results may be adversely affected. Examples of abnormal appearance that are discussed in more detail later in the course include:

Hemolyzed – Pink to red color, indicating red blood cell destruction

Icteric – Dark yellow color, indicating the presence of increased bilirubin

Lipemic – Cloudy, milky appearance, indicating the presence of increased lipids

Venous blood is the specimen of choice for clinical laboratory testing, and most normal values are based on venous blood. However, tests are also performed on arterial and capillary specimens. Arterial blood is the required specimen for arterial

Technical Tip

For anticoagulants to totally prevent clotting, specimens must be thoroughly mixed immediately following collection.

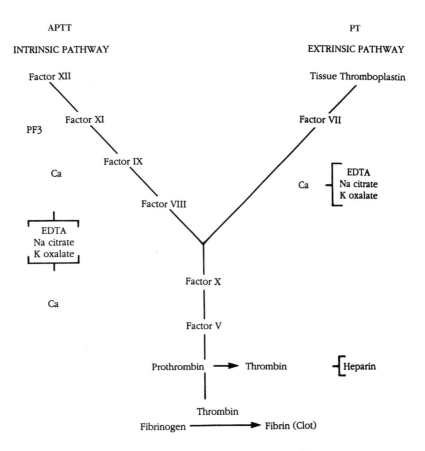

Figure 1-2

The role of anticoagulants in the coagulation cascade (Ca = calcium; PF3 = platelet factor 3)
(From Strasinger, SK, and Di Lorenzo, MA: Phlebotomy Workbook for the Multiskilled Healthcare Professional. FA Davis, Philadelphia, 1996, Figure 12-8, p. 180, with permission.)

blood gas determinations. In the interest of patient safety, only specifically trained personnel must perform arterial punctures. Arterial blood may also be collected from central lines.

Capillary blood is a mixture of arterial and venous blood and is collected by dermal puncture. When properly collected, capillary blood is suitable for many laboratory tests, but normal values may differ from those of venous blood. Therefore, requisition forms should indicate whether the specimen is arterial or capillary blood.

QUALITY ASSURANCE

Laboratory quality assurance is designed to guarantee quality patient care by ensuring accurate and reliable test results in an appropriate and timely manner. As can be seen from this brief introduction, many factors related to blood collection can affect laboratory quality assurance. These factors are covered in detail in the following units. In addition, remember that laboratory personnel are available to answer questions and should be consulted whenever necessary.

Venipuncture Equipment

Learning Objectives

Upon completion of this unit, the reader will be able to:

☐ Differentiate between an evacuated tube system, syringe, and a winged infusion set.

☐ Differentiate among the various needle sizes as to gauge and purpose.

☐ Discuss methods to safely dispose of contaminated needles.

☐ Identify the types of evacuated tubes by color code, and state the anticoagulants and additives present, the mechanism of action, any special characteristics, and the purpose of each.

☐ List the correct order of draw for the evacuated tube system and the correct order of fill for tubes collected by syringe.

☐ Discuss the purpose and types of tourniquets.

☐ Name two substances used to cleanse the skin prior to venipuncture.

☐ Discuss the use of gloves, sterile gauze, and bandages when performing venipuncture.

☐ Discuss the use of a blood collection tray, transport carriers, and drawing stations.

☐ Describe the quality control of venipuncture equipment.

INTRODUCTION

Considering the many types of blood specimens that may be required for laboratory testing and the risks to both patients and health-care personnel associated with blood collection, it is understandable that a considerable amount of equipment is required for the procedure.

This unit describes the various blood collection systems, collection tubes, order of draw, safety disposal systems, and other required supplies necessary for efficient blood collection.

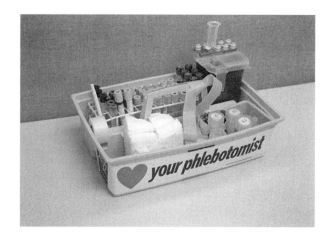

Figure 2–1

Blood collection tray
(From Strasinger, SK, and Di Lorenzo, MA: Phlebotomy Workbook for the Multi-skilled Healthcare Professional. FA Davis, Philadelphia, 1996, Figure 12-1, p. 174, with permission.)

ORGANIZATION OF EQUIPMENT

Technical Tip

A blood collector with well-organized equipment instills patient confidence.

An important key to successful blood collection is making sure that all the required equipment is conveniently present in the collection area. Trays designed to organize and transport collection equipment are available from several manufacturers (Figure 2–1). Maintaining a well-equipped blood collection tray that the blood collector carries into the patient's room (with the exception of isolation rooms) is the ideal way to prevent unnecessary errors during blood collection. Place the tray on a solid surface such as a nightstand and not on the patient's bed, where it can be knocked off. Trays should be emptied and disinfected on a weekly basis and more frequently if they become visibly soiled.

In outpatient settings, use a blood drawing chair with an attached or adjacently placed stand to hold equipment. Drawing chairs have an armrest that locks in place in front of the patient to provide arm support and protect the patient from falling out of the chair if he or she faints.

Venipuncture can be performed using an evacuated tube system, a syringe, or a winged infusion (butterfly) set. Each of these systems requires its own unique equipment, which is discussed in the following sections. Supplies that are common to all procedures are also discussed.

EVACUATED TUBE SYSTEM

The evacuated tube system (Figure 2–2) is the most frequently used method for performing venipuncture. Blood is collected directly into the evacuated tube, eliminating the need for transfer of specimens and minimizing the risk of biohazard exposure. The evacuated tube system consists of a double-pointed needle to puncture the stopper of the collection tube, an adapter to hold the needle and collection tube, and color-coded evacuated tubes, frequently referred to as Vacutainers (Becton Dickinson, Franklin Hills, NJ).

NEEDLES

Sterile needles for venipuncture are disposable and used only once. Needle size varies by both length and gauge. The needle gauge refers to the diameter of the needle; the

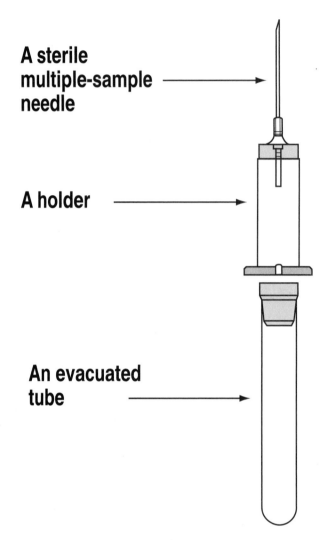

A sterile
multiple-sample
needle

A holder

An evacuated
tube

Figure 2–2

Evacuated tube
(From Wedding, ME, and
Toenjes, SA: Medical Labora-
tory Procedures, ed. 2.
FA Davis, Philadelphia, 1998,
p. 142, with permission.)

Technical Tip

**Many health-care work-
ers feel that they have
better control using
a 1-inch needle.**

lower the number, the larger the needle. The standard needles used with evacuated tubes are 20 to 22 gauge with a 1-inch or 1.5-inch length. Children and patients with small veins may require 23-gauge needles. Smaller evacuated tubes should be used with small-gauge needles because a small-diameter needle with a large evacuated tube can cause hemolysis. Needles used to collect units of blood for transfusion are the larger, 16-gauge needles.

Needles are packaged in sterile, twist-apart sealed shields that are color-coded according to the size of the needle and must not be used if the seal is broken. Needles used with an evacuated tube system are threaded in the middle and have a beveled point at each end. The front end is used to enter the vein, and the back end is used to penetrate the rubber stopper of an evacuated tube. A retractable rubber sheath covers the back end of the needle to prevent leakage of blood as tubes are changed or removed. Figure 2–3 shows the various needle structures. Needles should be visually examined for structural defects such as nonbeveled points or bent shafts immediately prior to use. Defective needles should not be used. Needles should never be recapped once the shield is removed regardless of whether they have or have not been used.

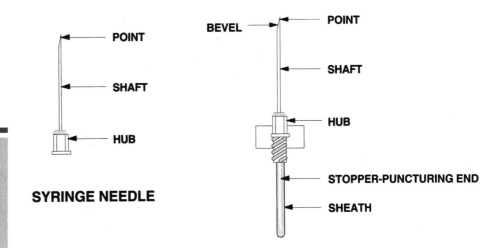

POINT

SHAFT

HUB

SYRINGE NEEDLE

BEVEL

POINT

SHAFT

HUB

STOPPER-PUNCTURING END

SHEATH

EVACUATED TUBE NEEDLE

Figure 2-3

Needle structures

(From Strasinger, SK, and Di Lorenzo, MA: Phlebotomy Workbook for the Multi-skilled Healthcare Professional. FA Davis, Philadelphia, 1996, Figure 12-3, p. 175, with permission.)

Many needles are currently equipped with safety shields and blunting devices. The Occupational Safety and Health Administration (OSHA) has issued a directive mandating the evaluation and implementation of safety devices. State mandates also have been issued. Safety shields covering the needles have been introduced with the SafetyGlide blood collection system (Becton Dickinson, Franklin Lakes, NJ). The blood collector pushes the movable shield along the cannula with the thumb to enclose the needle tip after venipuncture (Figure 2–4). The BD Vacutainer Eclipse blood collection needle utilizes a shield that the blood collector locks over the needle tip after completion of the venipuncture (Figure 2–5).

Self-blunting needles (Punctur-Guard by BioPlexus, Tolland, CT) are available to provide additional protection against needlestick injuries by making the needle blunt before removal from the patient. A hollow, blunt inner needle is contained inside the standard needle. Before removing the needle from the patient's vein, an additional push on the final tube in the adapter advances the internal blunt cannula past the sharp tip of the outer needle. The blunt cannula is hollow, allowing blood to continue to flow into the tube.

ADAPTERS/HOLDERS

Technical Tip

Loss of tube vacuum is a primary cause of failure to obtain blood. The venipuncture can be performed prior to placing the tube on the needle. Practice both methods and choose the one with which you are most comfortable.

Needle adapters used with evacuated collection systems are designed to accommodate different sizes of collection tubes. Adapters are made of clear, rigid plastic and are designed to act as a safety shield for the used needle.

The back end of the evacuated tube system needle screws securely onto the adapter. The first tube is partially advanced onto the stopper-puncturing needle up to a designated mark on the adapter. Pushing the tube beyond this point will break the tube's vacuum, making the tube unusable. The tube is fully advanced onto the end of the holder when the needle is in the vein. Blood will flow into the tube once the needle penetrates the stopper. The flared ends of the adapter aid the blood collector during the changing of tubes in multiple-draw situations (Figure 2–6). Tubes are removed with a slight twist to help disengage them from the needle.

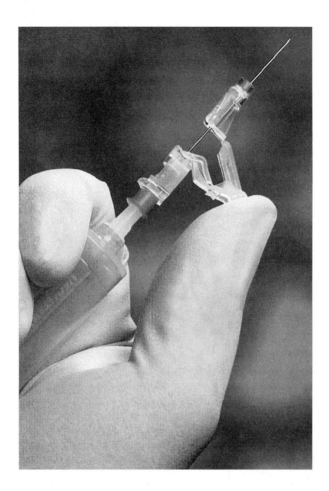

Figure 2–4

SafetyGlide blood collection assembly
(Courtesy of Becton Dickinson, Franklin Lakes, NJ.)

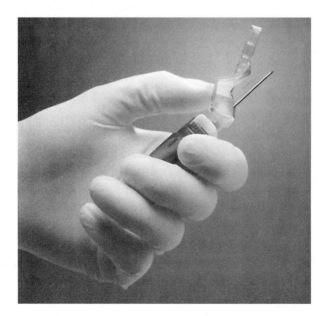

Figure 2–5

Eclipse blood collection needle with Pronto needle holder
(Courtesy of Becton Dickinson, Franklin Lakes, NJ.)

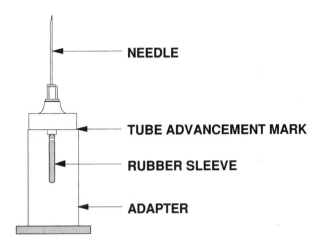

NEEDLE

TUBE ADVANCEMENT MARK

RUBBER SLEEVE

ADAPTER

Figure 2-6

Needle adapter
(From Strasinger, SK, and Di Lorenzo, MA: Phlebotomy Workbook for the Multi-skilled Healthcare Profes-sional. FA Davis, Philadel-phia, 1996, Figure 12-5, p. 177, with permission.)

NEEDLE DISPOSAL SYSTEMS

In June 2002, OSHA issued a revision to the Bloodborne Pathogens Standard compliance directive. In the revised directive, the agency requires that all blood holders (adapters) with needles attached be immediately discarded into a sharps container after the device's safety feature is activated. Rationale for the new directive is based on the exposure of workers to the unprotected stopper-puncturing end of evacuated tube needles, the increased needle manipulation required to remove it from the holder, and the possible worker exposure from the use of contaminated holders.

Safety adapters use a protective sleeve that is activated after use. Becton-Dickinson VACUTAINER System (Franklin Lakes, NJ) developed the Safety-Lok Needle Holder (Figure 2–7) with a splatter cap and a protective shield. The blood collector slides the shield over the needle and locks it in place after the needle is withdrawn from the vein, thus providing immediate containment of the used needle. The entire single-use device is disposed of in the sharps container. Needle-Pro (SIMS-Portex, Keene, NH) consists of a disposable plastic shield attached by a hinge to the end of the evacuated tube adapter. The shield hangs free during the venipuncture and is flipped over the needle using a single-handed technique after the puncture is performed. The entire device is discarded in the sharps container. The ProGuard II safety needle holder (Kendall Healthcare, Manchester, MA) provides a one-handed method to retract the needle into the holder and a cover for the end that is open to the stopper-puncturing needle (Figure 2-8).

A Portex Blood Draw Hypodermic Needle-Pro and the BD SafetyGlide hypodermic needle are available for syringe use (Figures 2-9 and 2-10).

Needles must always be placed in rigid, puncture-resistant, leak-proof dispos-able containers labeled BIOHAZARD that are easily sealed when full. Syringes with the needles attached, winged infusions sets, and adapters with needles attached are disposed of directly into puncture-resistant containers (Figure 2-11).

The BD blood transfer device (Becton, Dickinson, Franklin Lakes, NJ) provides a safer means for blood transfer when collecting blood with a syringe. It is an evacuated tube adapter with a rubber-sheathed needle inside. After blood collection, the syringe tip is inserted into the hub of the device and evacuated tubes are filled by pushing them onto the rubber-sheathed needle in the holder as in an evacuated tube system. The entire syringe/adapter assembly is discarded in the sharps container after use (Figure 2-12).

Technical Tip

To prevent accidental punctures from contami-nated needles, become thoroughly familiar with the operation of your needle safety sys-tem prior to perform-ing blood collection.

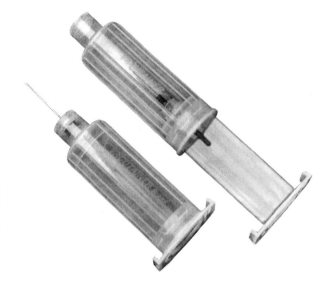

Figure 2-7

Safety-Lok needle holder
(Courtesy of Becton Dickinson, Franklin Lakes, NJ.)

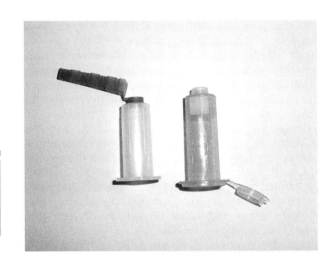

Figure 2-8

Portex Venipuncture Needle-Pro and Kendall ProGuard II safety needle holder.

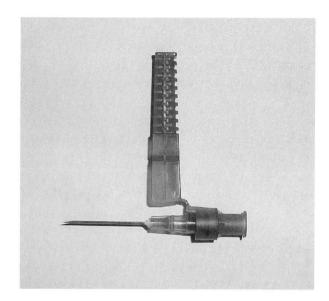

Figure 2–9

Portex Blood Draw Hypodermic Needle-Pro.
(Courtesy of Portex, Inc., Keene, NH.)

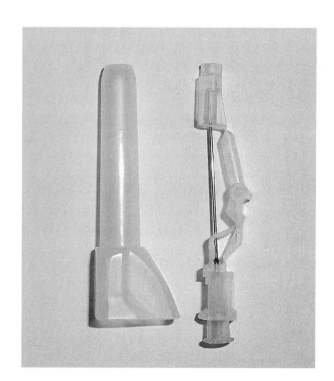

Figure 2–10

BD SafetyGlide™ hypodermic needle (safety device activated).
(Courtesy of Becton, Dickinson and Company © 2002 BD.)

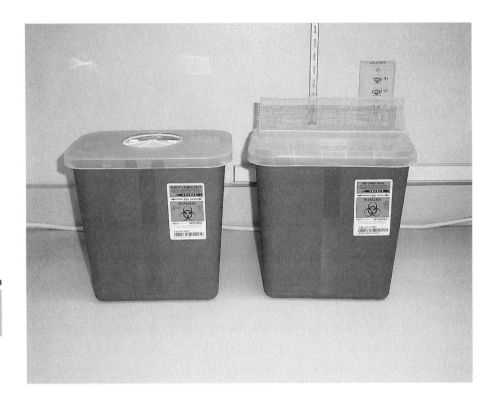

Figure 2-11

Sharps disposal containers.

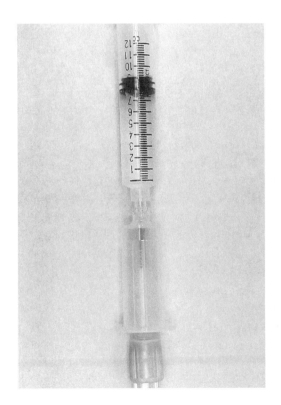

Figure 2-12

BD blood transfer device
(Courtesy of Becton, Dickinson and Company © 2002 BD.)

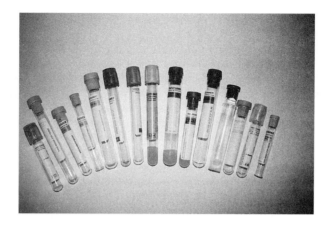

Figure 2-13

Examples of evacuated tubes

(From Strasinger, SK, and Di Lorenzo, MS: Skills for the Patient Care Technician. FA Davis, Philadelphia, 1999, Figure 5-6, p. 115, with permission.)

COLLECTION TUBES

The collection tubes used with the evacuated system (Figure 2–13) are available in glass and plastic and in a variety of sizes and volumes. The tubes are labeled with the type of anticoagulant or additive, the draw volume, and the expiration date. Evacuated tubes have color-coded rubber stoppers or plastic shields covering the rubber stoppers (Becton Dickinson Hemogard Vacutainer System, Franklin Lakes, NJ) to indicate the presence or absence of an additive or anticoagulant in the tube. The color-coding is universal and is used to describe the type of tube to use for sample collection, for example, "draw one red stopper and one light-blue stopper tube." This reference to tube color is found on most computer-generated requisition forms. Each laboratory department has specific specimen requirements for the analysis of particular blood constituents.

As shown in Figure 2–14, evacuated tubes have thick rubber stoppers with a

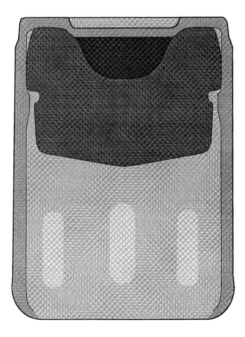

Figure 2-14

Cut-away view of a vacuum tube stopper (Hemogard closure)

(Adapted from product literature, Becton Dickinson, Franklin Lakes, NJ.)

thinner central area to allow puncture by the needle. Tubes may have a color-coded plastic safety shield covering the stopper to provide additional protection against blood splatter (Hemogard Vacutainer System) when stoppers are removed.

Evacuated tubes fill automatically because a premeasured vacuum is present in the tube. This causes some tubes to fill almost to the top, whereas other tubes only partially fill. Partial fill tubes have translucent colored Hemogard closures in the same color as regular fill tubes to distinguish them. The draw volume is written on the tube label. Most tubes are sterile and silicone coated to prevent cells from adhering to the wall of the tube, thereby decreasing hemolysis.

Tests requiring whole blood or plasma are collected in tubes containing an anticoagulant, which may be in a liquid or powder form. Different types of anticoagulants are required for specific tests. Prior to use, tubes with powdered anticoagulant should be gently tapped to loosen the powder for better mixing with the blood. All tubes containing an anticoagulant must be gently inverted 5 to 10 times immediately after collection to mix the contents and to avoid microclot formation. Tubes containing an anticoagulant must be completely filled to the designated volume draw. If the blood-to-anticoagulant ratio is incorrect, test results may be erroneous. Partial collection tubes should be used when a short draw is anticipated. Additives present in evacuated tubes are used as preservatives and clot activators. Tubes containing additives also must be gently mixed to ensure effectiveness. Blood collected in a tube containing an anticoagulant or additive cannot be transferred into a tube containing a different anticoagulant or additive.

Color-Coding of Tubes

Lavender stopper tubes and Hemogard closures contain the anticoagulant EDTA in the form of liquid tripotassium or spray-dried dipotassium ethylenediamine-tetraacetic acid. Coagulation is prevented by the binding of calcium in the specimen to sites on the large EDTA molecule, thereby preventing the participation of the calcium in the coagulation cascade (see Fig. 1–2). For hematology procedures that require whole blood, such as the complete blood count (CBC), EDTA is the anticoagulant of choice because it maintains cellular integrity better than other anticoagulants, inhibits platelet clumping, and does not interfere with routine staining procedures. In an underfilled EDTA tube, the excess anticoagulant may shrink red blood cells and affect hematology tests. However, the tubes can be submitted to the laboratory for evaluation if necessary. Lavender stopper tubes cannot be used for coagulation studies because EDTA interferes with factor V and the thrombin-fibrinogen reaction.

Light-blue stopper tubes and Hemogard closures contain the anticoagulant sodium citrate, which also prevents coagulation by binding calcium. Centrifugation of the anticoagulated light-blue stopper tubes provides the plasma used for coagulation tests. Sodium citrate is the required anticoagulant for coagulation studies because it preserves the labile coagulation factors.

The ratio of blood to the liquid sodium citrate is critical and should be 9:1 (example: 4.5 mL blood and 0.5 mL sodium citrate). This tube requires a full draw to prevent dilution of coagulation factors. When drawing coagulation tests on patients with polycythemia or hematocrit readings over 55 percent, the amount of anticoagulant must be decreased to maintain the 9:1 ratio, because the lower volume of plasma in these patients will be diluted by the standard volume of sodium citrate. Likewise, the amount of anticoagulant must be increased for severely anemic patients because of the larger amount of plasma. The laboratory should be consulted to provide tubes with the appropriate amount of anticoagulant.

A special light-blue stopper tube containing thrombin and a soybean trypsin inhibitor must be used when drawing blood for determinations of certain fibrin degradation products.

Technical Tip

The laboratory always rejects incompletely filled light-blue stopper tubes.

Black stopper tubes containing sodium citrate are used for Westergren sedimentation rates. They differ from light-blue stopper tubes in that they provide a ratio of blood to liquid anticoagulant of 4:1. Specially designed tubes for Westergren sedimentation rates are available.

Green stopper tubes and Hemogard closures contain the anticoagulant heparin combined with sodium, lithium, or ammonium ion. Heparin prevents clotting by inhibiting thrombin in the coagulation cascade (see Fig. 1–2). Green stopper tubes are used for chemistry tests performed on plasma including ammonia, carboxyhemoglobin, and stat electrolytes. Interference by sodium and lithium heparin with their corresponding chemical tests and by ammonium heparin in blood urea nitrogen (BUN) determinations must be avoided. Green stopper tubes are not used for hematology because heparin interferes with the Wright's stained blood smear used for differentials.

Light-green Hemogard closure tubes and **green/black** stopper tubes contain lithium heparin and a separation gel and are called plasma separator tubes (PST). PST tubes are used for plasma determinations in chemistry. They are well suited for potassium determinations because heparin prevents the release of potassium by platelets during clotting and the gel prevents contamination of the plasma by red blood cell potassium.

Yellow/gray rubber stoppers and **orange Hemogard closures** are found on tubes containing the clot activator thrombin. The addition of thrombin to the tube results in faster clot formation, usually within 5 minutes. Tubes containing thrombin are used for stat serum chemistry determinations and on samples from patients receiving anticoagulant therapy.

Gray stopper tubes and Hemogard closures are available with a variety of additives and anticoagulants for the primary purpose of preserving glucose. All gray stopper tubes contain a glucose preservative (antiglycolytic agent), either sodium fluoride or lithium iodoacetate. Sodium fluoride maintains glucose for 3 days and iodoacetate for 24 hours. Sodium fluoride and iodoacetate are not anticoagulants; therefore, if plasma is needed for analysis, anticoagulant must also be present. In gray stopper tubes, the anticoagulant is potassium oxalate, which, like EDTA and sodium citrate, prevents clotting by binding calcium. When monitoring patient glucose levels, tubes for the collection of plasma and serum should not be interchanged. Gray stopper tubes should not be used for other chemical analyses because sodium fluoride interferes with some enzyme analyses. Gray stopper tubes are not used in hematology because oxalate distorts cellular morphology.

Blood alcohol levels are drawn in gray top tubes containing sodium fluoride because microbial growth, which could produce alcohol as a metabolic end product, is inhibited. Tubes with or without potassium oxalate can be used, depending on the need for plasma or serum in the test procedure.

Royal blue stopper tubes and Hemogard closures are used for trace elements, toxicology, and nutrient determinations. Because many of the elements analyzed in these studies are significant at very low levels, the tubes must be chemically clean, and the rubber stoppers are specially formulated to contain the lowest possible levels of metal. Royal blue stopper tubes are available plain or with sodium heparin or EDTA to conform to a variety of testing requirements.

Brown Hemogard closure tubes are available for lead determinations. They are certified to contain less than 0.01 μg/mL (ppm) lead.

Yellow stopper tubes are available for two different purposes and contain different additives. Yellow stoppers and yellow Hemogard closures are found on tubes containing the red blood cell preservative acid citrate dextrose (ACD). Specimens collected in these tubes are used for special cellular studies in the blood bank.

Figure 2-15

Serum separator tubes before and after collection and centrifugation
(From Strasinger, SK, and Di Lorenzo, MA: Phlebotomy Workbook for the Multi-skilled Healthcare Professional. FA Davis, Philadelphia, 1996, Figure 12-9, p. 181, with permission.)

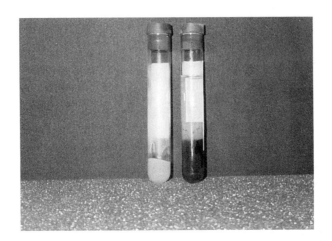

Technical Tip

Centrifugation of incompletely clotted SST tubes can produce a nonintact gel barrier and possible cellular contamination of the serum.

Sterile **yellow** stopper tubes containing the anticoagulant sodium polyanetholesulfonate (SPS) are used to collect specimens to be cultured for the presence of microorganisms. SPS aids in the recovery of microorganisms by inhibiting the actions of complement, phagocytes, and certain antibiotics.

Red/gray rubber stoppers and **gold Hemogard closures** are found on tubes containing a clot activator and a separation gel. They are referred to as serum separator tubes (SST). The tubes contain silica that increases platelet activation, thereby shortening the time required for clot formation. Tubes should be inverted five times to expose the blood to the clot activator. A nonreactive thixotropic gel that undergoes a temporary change in viscosity during centrifugation is located at the bottom of the tube. As shown in Figure 2–15, when the tube is centrifuged, the gel forms a barrier between the cells and serum to prevent contamination of the serum with cellular materials. To produce a solid separation barrier, specimens must be allowed to clot completely before centrifuging. Specimens should be centrifuged as soon as clot formation is complete, which is usually about 10 to 15 minutes. Serum separator tubes are used for most chemistry tests. They prevent contamination of the serum by cellular chemicals and products of cellular metabolism. They are not suitable for blood bank and certain immunology/serology tests.

Red stopper glass tubes and Hemogard closures are often referred to as plain or clot tubes because they contain no anticoagulants or additives. Blood drawn in red stopper tubes clots by the normal coagulation process in about 30 minutes. Centrifugation of the specimen then yields serum as the liquid portion. Red stopper tubes are used for serum chemistry tests, serology tests, and in blood bank, where both serum and red blood cells may be used. There is no need to invert red stopper tubes.

Notice the emphasis placed on glass red stopper tubes. Plastic red stopper tubes are also available, and these tubes contain silica as a clot activator. They are used for the same purpose as the glass tubes and are inverted to initiate the clotting process.

Appendix 3 summarizes evacuated tubes and their uses.

ORDER OF DRAW

Often several tests are ordered on patients, and blood must be collected in different tubes. The order in which tubes are drawn is one of the most important considerations when collecting blood specimens, as this can affect some test results. Tubes must be collected in a specific order to prevent invalid test results caused by contamination of the specimen by tissue fluid or carry-over of additives or anticoagulants between tubes.

For example, the release of tissue thromboplastin from the skin as it is punctured can result in its presence in the first tube collected, and this could interfere with coagulation tests. Therefore, a light-blue stopper tube should not be drawn first. If only a coagulation test is ordered, it is recommended that a small red stopper tube be drawn first and then discarded. Recent studies suggest that the discard tube may no longer be necessary for routine coagulation tests (activated partial thromboplastin time [APTT] and prothrombin time [PT]), but it is still required for special coagulation tests. It is important that the blood collector follow the blood collection protocol of the facility.

Transfer of anticoagulants when changing tubes as a result of possible contamination of the stopper-puncturing needle must be avoided. This is why the nonadditive red stopper tube is drawn before the coagulation tube and why tubes containing anticoagulants are drawn after the light-blue stopper tube. When one considers the mechanisms of anticoagulation and the chemical composition of the various anticoagulants, it can be understood that the results of several frequently requested tests could be compromised by contamination. For example, contamination of a green or red stopper tube designated for sodium, potassium, and calcium determinations with EDTA, sodium citrate, or potassium oxalate would falsely decrease the calcium and elevate the sodium or potassium results. Holding blood collection tubes in a downward position helps avoid the transfer of anticoagulants from tube to tube.

When sterile specimens, such as blood cultures, are to be collected, they must be considered in the order of draw. Such specimens are always drawn first to prevent contamination.

Recommendations for the order of draw vary slightly between manufacturers, the National Committee on Clinical Laboratory Standards (NCCLS), and individual laboratories. Laboratory protocol should be followed for this placement.

The following summary of the order of draw recommended by NCCLS can be used as a guideline:

- Sterile specimens (yellow, culture bottles)
- Red glass stopper tubes (plain, no additive)
- Light-blue stopper tubes (sodium citrate)
- Red/gray SST, gold SST, and red plastic stopper tubes (clot activator)
- Green stopper tubes and light green PST tubes (heparin)
- Lavender stopper tubes (EDTA)
- Gray stopper tubes (oxalate, fluoride)
- Yellow/gray or orange stopper tubes (thrombin clot activator)

SYRINGES

Syringes may be preferred over an evacuated tube system when drawing blood from patients with small or fragile veins. The advantage of this system is that the amount of suction pressure on the vein can be controlled by slowly pulling back the syringe plunger.

Figure 2-16

Diagram of a syringe.
(From Strasinger, SK, and
Di Lorenzo, MA: Phlebotomy
Workbook for the Multi-
skilled Healthcare Professional. FA Davis, Philadelphia, 1996, Figure 12-10,
p. 184, with permission.)

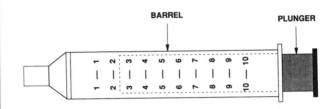

Syringes consist of a barrel graduated in milliliters (mL) or cubic centimeters (cc) and a plunger that fits tightly within the barrel creating a vacuum when retracted (Figure 2–16). Syringes used for venipuncture range from 2 to 10 mL, and the blood collector should use a size that corresponds to the amount of blood needed. Needles are attached to a plastic hub designed to fit on the barrel of the syringe. The technique for use of syringes is discussed in Unit 4.

Syringes that provide a protective sheath to cover the needle before disposal are available. Disposable plastic sheaths that are attached to the end of a syringe can be flipped up over the needle after use (Vacu-Pro Needle Clip, Sims/Smith Industries, Keene, NH).

Blood drawn in a syringe must be immediately transferred to appropriate evacuated tubes to prevent the formation of clots. Blood is transferred by puncturing the rubber stopper with the syringe needle and allowing the blood to be drawn, but not forced, into the tube. To prevent hemolysis, the needle should be angled toward the side of the tube for gentler transfer of the blood. Care must be taken to avoid needle punctures. As shown in Figure 2–17, the tube should be placed in a rack, not held in the free hand.

When tubes are filled from a syringe, NCCLS recommends that tubes be filled in the same order as recommended for the order of draw previously listed. Some

Technical Tip

Let the vacuum in the evacuated tube draw the appropriate amount of blood into the tube. Discard any extra blood left in the syringe, do not force it into the tube.

Figure 2-17

Transfer of blood from a syringe to an evac-uated tube. (Note how the collector directs the blood against the side of the tube.)
(From Strasinger, SK, and
Di Lorenzo, MA: Phlebotomy
Workbook for the Multi-
skilled Healthcare Professional. FA Davis, Philadelphia, 1996, Figure 12-11,
p. 185, with permission.)

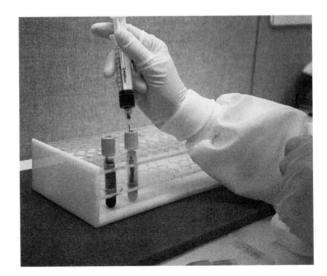

institutions, however, feel that because the portion of blood possibly contaminated by tissue thromboplastin is the first portion to enter the syringe, it is the last to be expelled. At these institutions, the order of transfer should be:

- Sterile specimens
- Light-blue stopper tubes
- Other anticoagulants and additives
  - Lavender stopper tube
  - Green stopper tube
  - Gray stopper tube
- Red and red/gray or orange stopper tubes

Institutional policy should be followed.

WINGED INFUSION SETS

Winged infusion sets, or butterflies as they are routinely called, are used for:

- The infusion of IV fluids
- Performing venipuncture from very small veins
- Obtaining specimens from children

Butterfly needles used for phlebotomy are usually 23-gauge with lengths of ½ to ¾ inch. Plastic attachments to the needle, which resemble butterfly wings, are used for holding the needle during insertion and to secure the apparatus during IV therapy (Figure 2–18). They also provide the ability to lower the needle insertion angle when working with very small veins. To accommodate the dual purpose of

Figure 2-18

Winged infusion set

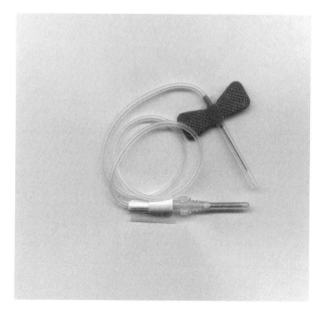

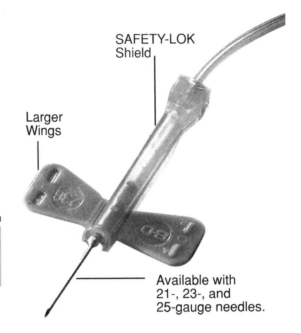

SAFETY-LOK
Shield

Larger
Wings

Figure 2-19

Safety-Lok blood col-
lection set
(Courtesy of Becton Dickinson, Franklin Lakes, NJ.)

Available with
21-, 23-, and
25-gauge needles.

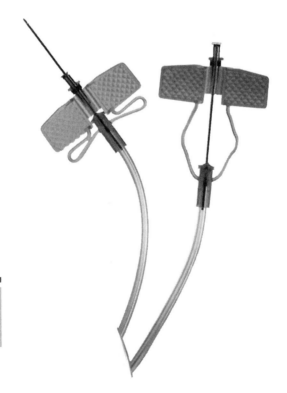

Figure 2-20

Angel Wing safety
needles
(Courtesy of Kendall,
Mansfield, MA.)

venipuncture and infusion, the needle is attached to a flexible plastic tubing that can be attached to an IV set-up, syringe, or specially designed evacuated tube adapters. Extreme care must be taken when working with winged infusion sets to avoid accidental needle punctures.

There are several winged needle sets with safety devices built into the system. The Vacutainer Safety-Lok (Becton Dickinson) uses a retractable safety enclosure that covers the needle once it has been withdrawn. After use, the needle is completely retracted into the protective shield and locked in place by pushing the yellow shield forward (Figure 2–19). Another widely used needle set is the Angel Wing safety needle (Kendall, Mansfield, MA) (Figure 2–20). When the needle is withdrawn, a stainless steel safety shield is activated and locks in place to cover the needle. The Puncture Guard winged infusion set (Bio-Plexus, Tolland, CT) produces a safety device that blunts the needle before withdrawal from the vein.

The technique for the use of winged infusion sets is covered in Unit 4.

TOURNIQUETS

Tourniquets are used during venipuncture to make it easier to locate patients veins. They do this by impeding venous, but not arterial, blood flow in the area just below the tourniquet application site. The distended vein then becomes more visible or palpable.

The most frequently used tourniquets are flat latex strips (Figure 2–21). They are inexpensive and may be disposed of between patients or reused if disinfected. Tourniquets with Velcro and buckle closures are easier to apply but are more difficult to decontaminate. Rubber tubing may be used for pediatric patients. Flat nonlatex strips are available for persons allergic to latex.

Blood pressure cuffs can be used as tourniquets. The cuff should be inflated to a pressure below the patient's systolic blood pressure reading and above the diastolic reading to allow blood to flow into but not out of the affected veins. The application of tourniquets and the effects on blood tests are discussed in Units 3 and 4.

Figure 2-21

Flat latex strip tourniquet
(From Strasinger, SK, and Di Lorenzo, MA: Phlebotomy Workbook for the Multi-skilled Healthcare Professional. FA Davis, Philadelphia, 1996, Figure 12–13, p. 186, with permission.)

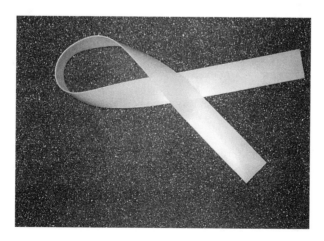

GLOVES

OSHA mandates that gloves must be worn when collecting blood and must be changed after each patient. Under routine circumstances, gloves do not need to be sterile. To provide maximal manual dexterity, they should fit securely.

Gloves are available in several varieties, including powdered and powder-free and latex and nonlatex. Allergy to latex is increasing among health-care workers. Persons developing symptoms of allergy to latex should avoid latex gloves and other latex products, such as tourniquets, at all times.

ANTISEPTICS

The recommended antiseptic used for cleansing the skin in routine blood collection is 70 percent isopropyl alcohol. This is a bacteriostatic antiseptic used to prevent contamination by normal skin bacteria during the short period required to perform collection of the specimen. Individually wrapped prep pads are available for convenience.

For collections that require additional sterility, such as blood cultures and arterial punctures, stronger antiseptics, including iodine or chlorhexidine gluconate (for patients allergic to iodine), are used to cleanse the area. To prevent skin discomfort, iodine should always be removed from the patient's skin with alcohol after a collection procedure.

GAUZE/BANDAGES

Sterile 2 × 2–inch gauze pads are used for applying pressure to the puncture site immediately after the needle has been removed. Gauze pads can also provide additional pressure when folded in quarters and placed under a bandage. Bandages or adhesive tape are placed over the puncture site when the bleeding has stopped. Patients should be instructed to remove the bandage within 1 hour.

ADDITIONAL SUPPLIES

An essential piece of equipment is a pen for labeling tubes, initialing computer-generated labels, or noting unusual circumstances on the requisition form. Biohazard bags should be available for transport of specimens based on institutional protocol.

QUALITY CONTROL

Ensuring the sterility of needles and puncture devices and the stability of evacuated tubes, anticoagulants, and additives is essential to patient safety and specimen quality. Disposable needles and puncture devices are individually packaged in tightly sealed sterile containers. Blood collectors should not use puncture equipment if the seal has been broken. Visual inspection for nonpointed or barbed needles may detect manufacturing defects.

Manufacturers of evacuated tubes must ensure that tubes, anticoagulants, and additives meet the standards established by the NCCLS. Evacuated tubes produced at the same time are referred to as a lot and have a distinguishing lot number printed on the packages. There is also an expiration date printed on each package. The expiration date represents the last day the manufacturer guarantees the stability of the specified amount of vacuum in the tube and the reactivity of the anticoagulants and additives. The expiration date should be checked each time a new package of tubes is opened, and outdated tubes should not be used. Use of expired tubes may cause incompletely filled tubes (short draws), clotted anticoagulated specimens, improperly preserved specimens, and insecure gel barriers.

Failure to completely fill tubes (short draws) containing anticoagulants and additives affects specimen quality because the amount of anticoagulant or additive present in the tube is based on the assumption that the tube will be completely filled. Possible errors include excessive dilution of the specimen by liquid anticoagulants and distortion of cellular structures by increased chemical concentrations.

Venipuncture Equipment Selection   *Exercise*

Instructions: State or assemble (if requested) the appropriate equipment for the following situations. Include the number and color of evacuated tubes; needle size, syringe size, or butterfly, if appropriate. Instructors may specify the inclusion of supplies.

1. Collection of a CBC specimen from a 35-year-old woman.

2. Collection of a CBC specimen from a 3-year-old boy.

3. Collection of specimens for a stat CBC and electrolytes from a 40-year-old man.

4. Collection of a cholesterol specimen from the hand of an obese patient.

5. Collection of a specimen for a coagulation test from an elderly patient.

6. Assemble the equipment to collect a specimen for a type and cross-match on a 50-year-old man.

_____

_____

_____

7. Assemble the equipment to collect a specimen for a cardiac risk profile and a prothrombin time from a patient with fragile veins.

_____

_____

_____

Routine Venipuncture

Upon completion of this unit, the reader will be able to:

☐ List the required information on a requisition form.

☐ Describe correct patient identification and specimen labeling procedures.

☐ Describe patient preparation and the variables that can affect some laboratory tests.

☐ Correctly assemble venipuncture equipment and supplies.

☐ Name and locate the three most frequently used veins for venipuncture, and describe when these sites would be unacceptable.

☐ Correctly apply a tourniquet and state why the tourniquet can be applied for only 1 minute.

☐ List four methods used to locate veins that are not prominent.

☐ Describe the different antiseptics used to cleanse the venipuncture site.

☐ State the steps in a venipuncture procedure, and correctly perform a routine venipuncture using an evacuated tube system.

☐ Demonstrate safe disposal of contaminated needles and supplies.

☐ Deliver specimens to the laboratory in a timely manner.

INTRODUCTION

The venipuncture technique consists of a series of steps that, when practiced consistently, provide quality specimens and cause minimal patient discomfort. Administrative protocols vary among institutions, and, of course, every patient is different; however, many basic rules are the same in all situations. These basic rules must be followed to ensure the safety of the patient and the person performing the procedure and to produce specimens that are representative of the patient's condition.

This unit presents a detailed description of the recommended steps in the venipuncture procedure and possible complications that could occur at each step.

BLOOD COLLECTION PROCEDURE

EXAMINE THE REQUISITION FORM

Technical Tip

Personnel should never collect samples prior to generating the requisition form.

All blood collection procedures begin with the receipt of a test requisition form generated by or at the request of a health-care provider. The requisition is essential to provide the blood collector with the information needed to correctly identify the patient, organize the necessary equipment, collect the appropriate specimens, and provide legal protection. Blood specimens should not be collected without a requisition form, and this form must accompany the specimens sent to the laboratory.

The actual format of a requisition form may vary. Patient information may be handwritten or imprinted on color-coded forms with test check-off lists for different departments. There may be multiple copies for purposes of record keeping and billing. Computer-generated forms may include not only the patient information and tests requested but also the tube labels and bar codes for specimen processing, the number and type of collection tubes needed, and special collection instructions.

When working in emergency care, a preprinted requisition form may not be available, making it necessary for the information to be written on a blank form. Be sure to transfer the identification number from the patient's wristband when a temporary identification system has been used. When verbal orders are given, the name of the person giving the order should be documented.

Requisitions must contain certain basic information to ensure that the specimen drawn and the test results are correlated to the appropriate patient and the results can be correctly interpreted with regard to any special conditions, such as the time of collection. The information includes the following:

1. Patient's name and identification number
2. Accession number
3. Patient's location
4. Health-care provider's name
5. Tests requested
6. Date and time of specimen collection

Other information that may be present includes:

- Patient's date of birth
- Special collection information (such as fasting specimen)
- Special patient information (such as areas that should not be used for venipuncture)
- Number and type of collection tubes
- Status of specimen (such as stat or preoperative)

GREET THE PATIENT

The blood collector should introduce himself or herself and explain that he or she will be collecting a blood specimen. Whenever possible, patients who are sleeping should be awakened and allowed to orient themselves prior to the procedure.

Unconscious patients should be greeted in the same manner as conscious patients, because they may be capable of hearing and understanding even though they cannot respond. In this circumstance, it may be necessary to request assistance from other members of the unit staff, because the patient may move when the needle is inserted.

IDENTIFY THE PATIENT

The most important step in the venipuncture procedure is the correct identification of the patient. Serious diagnostic or treatment errors and even death can occur when blood is drawn from the wrong patient.

To ensure that blood is drawn from the right patient, compare the information obtained verbally and from the patient's wrist identification (ID) band with the information on the requisition. A wristband lying on the bedside table cannot be used for identification because it could belong to anyone. Likewise, a sign over the patient's bed or on the door cannot be relied on for identification because the patient could be in the wrong bed or room.

Verbal identification is made after the patient greeting by asking the patient to state his or her full name. In an outpatient setting, comparison of verbal information with the requisition form may be the only means of verifying identification. Asking patients for their date of birth or asking them to spell their last name may be helpful in this situation. Do not ask, " Are you Mr. Jones?" because many patients will say "yes" to any questions asked. Verify that the computer-generated sample labels match the requisition and patient identification.

For inpatients, examining the information on the patient's wristband, which should be present on all hospitalized patients, follows verbal identification. All information on the wrist ID band must match the information on the requisition form. The information should be identical, and any discrepancies investigated prior to obtaining the specimen.

Patients without ID bands attached to their bodies should be rebanded according to unit procedures prior to specimen collection. The name of the person identifying the patient should be documented.

Unidentified patients are sometimes brought into the emergency room, and a system must be in place to ensure they are correctly matched with their laboratory work. The American Association of Blood Banks requires that the patient is positively identified with a temporary but clear designation attached to the body. Some hospitals generate ID bands with an ID number and a tentative name, such as John Doe, or Patient X. Commercial identification systems are particularly useful when blood transfusions are required. In these systems, the ID band that is attached to the patient comes with matching identification stickers. The stickers are placed on the specimen tubes, the requisition form, and any units of blood designated for the patient. Blood bank identification systems are used in addition to routine ID bands, not instead of them.

Technical Tip

Personnel already familiar with a patient must never become lax with regard to patient identification.

PREPARE THE PATIENT

The patient must be positioned conveniently and safely for the procedure. Provide a brief explanation of the procedure, but do not discuss the actual tests that are to be performed. Patients should not be told that the procedure will be painless.

While talking with the patient, verify that any pretest preparation, such as fasting or abstaining from medications, has occurred. When these procedures have not been followed and the specimen is still required, the irregular condition, such as nonfasting, should be noted on the requisition form and on the specimen.

Numerous variables associated with a patient's activities prior to specimen collection can affect the quality of the specimen. These variables can include diet,

Table 3-1 Major Tests Affected by Patient Variables

Variable	Increased Results	Decreased Results
Nonfasting	Glucose and triglycerides	
Prolonged fasting	Bilirubin, fatty acids, and triglycerides	Glucose
Posture	Albumin, bilirubin, calcium, enzymes, lipids, total protein, RBCs, and WBCs	
Short-term exercise	Creatinine, fatty acids, lactate, AST, CK, LD, and WBCs	
Long-term exercise	Aldolase, creatinine, sex hormones, AST, CK, and LD	
Stress	Adrenal hormones, fatty acids, lactate, and WBCs	
Alcohol	Lactate, triglycerides, uric acid, GGT, HDL, and MCV	
Tobacco	Catecholamines, cortisol, hemoglobin, MCV, and WBCs	
Diurnal variation (AM)	Cortisol, serum iron	WBCs

AST, aspartate aminotransferase; CK, creatine kinase; GGT, gamma-glutamyl transpeptidase; HDL, high-density lipoprotein; LD, lactate dehydrogenase; MCV, mean corpuscular volume; RBCs, red blood cells; WBCs, white blood cells.

posture, exercise, stress, alcohol, smoking, time of day, and medications. Major tests affected by these variables are listed in Table 3–1.

To guard against a possible episode of syncope, patients should always be sitting or lying down when phlebotomy is performed. Never draw blood from a patient who is standing. Outpatients should be seated at a drawing station, preferably one with a movable arm that serves the dual purpose of providing a solid surface for the patient's arm and preventing a patient who faints from falling out of the chair. Patients who have had previous difficulties during venipuncture should lie down for the procedure. Placing a pillow or towel under the patient's arm can provide comfortable support. Asking the patient to make a fist with the opposite hand and place it behind the elbow will provide support. The arm should be firmly supported and extended downward in a straight line, allowing the tube to fill from the bottom up to prevent reflux and anticoagulant carryover between sample tubes.

Patients should remove any object, such as gum or a thermometer, from their mouth before performance of the venipuncture.

Technical Tip

Patients are often more comfortable if gloves are donned in their presence, which reassures them that sterility is being maintained.

WASH HANDS AND APPLY GLOVES

Always apply clean gloves between each patient, and wash hands before and after the procedure. Pull gloves over the cuffs of protective clothing.

SELECT EQUIPMENT

Before approaching the patient for the actual venipuncture, the blood collector should collect all necessary supplies (including collection equipment, antiseptic pads, sterile gauze, bandages, and needle disposal system) and place them close to the patient. Reexamine the requisition form, and select the appropriate number and type of collection tubes. Place the tubes in the correct order for specimen collection,

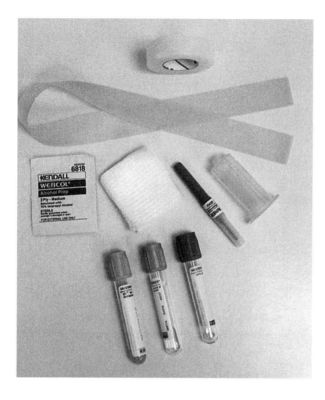

Figure 3–1

Venipuncture collection equipment

(From Strasinger, SK, and Di Lorenzo, MS: Skills for the Patient Care Technician. FA Davis, Philadelphia, 1999, Figure 6–4, p. 139, with permission.)

and have additional tubes readily available for possible use during the procedure (Figure 3–1). It is not uncommon to find a vacuum tube that does not contain the necessary amount of vacuum to collect a full tube of blood. Accidentally pushing a tube past the indicator mark on the adapter before the vein is entered also results in loss of vacuum.

APPLY THE TOURNIQUET

The tourniquet serves two functions in the venipuncture procedure. By causing blood to accumulate in the veins, the tourniquet causes the veins to be more easily located and also provides a larger amount of blood for collection. Use of a tourniquet can alter some test results by increasing the ratio of cellular elements to plasma (hemoconcentration) and by causing hemolysis. Therefore, the maximum time a tourniquet should remain in place is 1 minute. This may require that the tourniquet be applied twice during the venipuncture procedure; first when vein selection is being made and then immediately before the puncture is performed. When the tourniquet is used during vein selection, it should be released for 2 minutes before being reapplied.

Tests most likely to be affected by prolonged tourniquet application are those measuring large molecules, such as plasma proteins and lipids or analytes affected by hemolysis, including potassium, lactic acid, and enzymes. During multiple tube collections, the tourniquet must be removed when the timing exceeds 1 minute. Tourniquet application and fist clenching are not recommended when drawing specimens for lactic acid determinations.

Ideally the tourniquet should be released as soon as blood begins to flow into the first tube to prevent hemoconcentration and hemolysis. Difficulty filling additional tubes may be encountered, however; the tourniquet may have to be retightened or pressure applied to the area with the free hand to increase the amount of blood present in the vein.

The tourniquet should be placed on the arm 3 to 4 inches above the venipuncture site. Application of the commonly used latex strip requires practice to develop a smooth technique and can be difficult if properly fitting gloves are not worn. Figure 3–2 shows the technique used with latex strip tourniquets. To achieve adequate pressure, both sides of the tourniquet must be grasped near the patient's arm, and while maintaining tension, the left side is tucked under the right side. The loop formed should face downward. The free ends of the tourniquet must be pointing away from the venipuncture site to avoid contaminating the site and must be able to be easily released with one hand. Left-handed persons would reverse this procedure.

Tourniquets that are folded or applied too tightly are uncomfortable for the patient and may obstruct blood flow to the area. The appearance of small, reddish discolorations (petechiae) on the patient's arm, blanching of the skin around the

Figure 3-2

Tourniquet application. *A*, Position the latex strip 3 to 4 inches above the venipuncture site. *B*, Cross the tourniquet over the patient's arm. *C*, Hold the tourniquet in one hand close to the arm. *D*, Tuck a portion of one end under the opposite end to form a loop. *E*, Properly applied tourniquet. *F*, Pull end of loop to release tourniquet.

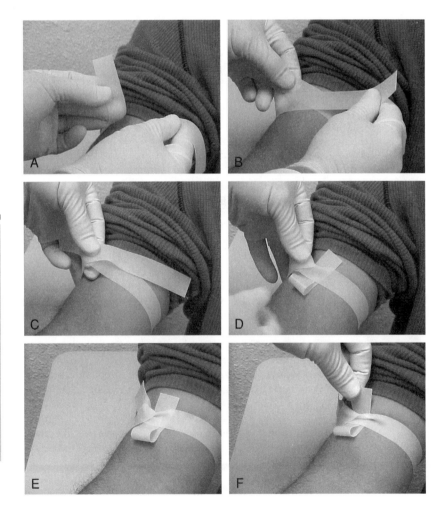

tourniquet, and the blood collector's inability to feel a radial pulse are indications of a tourniquet tied too tightly.

When dealing with patients with skin conditions or open sores, it may be necessary to place the tourniquet over the patient's gown or to cover the area with gauze prior to application. If possible, another area should be selected for the venipuncture. Consideration should also be given to using a disposable tourniquet. Do not apply a tourniquet to an arm on the same side as a mastectomy.

SELECT THE VENIPUNCTURE SITE

Technical Tip

When supporting the patient's arm, do not hyperextend the elbow. This may make vein palpation difficult. Sometimes bending the elbow very slightly may aid in vein palpation.

The preferred site for venipuncture is the antecubital fossa located anterior to the elbow. As shown in Figure 3–3, the median cubital, cephalic, and basilic veins are located in this area, and in most patients at least one of these veins can be easily located. Notice that the veins continue down the forearm to the wrist area; however, in these areas the veins become smaller and less well anchored, and punctures are more painful to the patient. Small, prominent veins are also located in the back of the hand. When necessary, these veins can be used for venipuncture but may require a smaller needle or butterfly set. The veins of the lower arm and hand are also the preferred sites for administering IV fluids because they allow the patient more arm flexibility. Frequent venipuncture in these veins could make them unsuitable for IV use. Some institutions have special ID bands that indicate the restricted use of veins being used for other procedures.

Of the three veins located in the antecubital area, the median cubital is the vein of choice because it is large, well anchored, and does not tend to move when the needle is inserted. It is often closer to the surface of the skin, more isolated from underlying structures, and the least painful to puncture. The cephalic vein located on the thumb side of the arm is usually more difficult to locate, except possibly in obese patients, and has more tendency to move. The cephalic vein should be the second

Figure 3–3

The veins in the arm most often chosen for venipuncture
(From Strasinger, SK, and Di Lorenzo, MA: Phlebotomy Workbook for the Multi-skilled Healthcare Professional. FA Davis, Philadelphia, 1996, Figure 13–6, p. 204, with permission.)

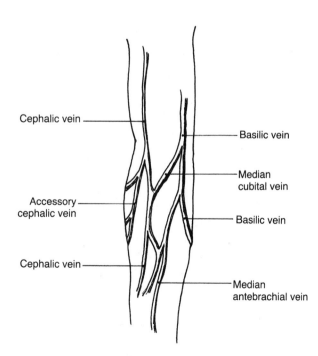

Cephalic vein

Basilic vein

Median cubital vein

Accessory cephalic vein

Basilic vein

Cephalic vein

Median antebrachial vein

Technical Tip

Patients often think they are helping by pumping their fists, because this is an acceptable practice when donating blood. In contrast to laboratory specimens, a donated unit of blood is even better when it is hemoconcentrated.

Technical Tip

Using the nondominant hand for palpation may be helpful when additional palpation is to be done immediately before performing the puncture.

Technical Tip

To increase the sensitivity of the palpating finger when wearing gloves, swab the finger with alcohol. Do not make a hole in the glove finger.

Technical Tip

Never be reluctant to check both arms and to listen to the patient's suggestions.

choice if the median cubital is inaccessible in both arms. The basilic vein is the least firmly anchored and is located near the brachial artery. Care must be taken not to accidentally puncture the artery. The basilic vein should be used as the last choice because the median nerve and brachial artery are in close proximity to it, increasing the risk of injury. Only superficial veins should be used in children.

Two routine steps in the venipuncture procedure aid in locating a suitable vein: applying a tourniquet and asking the patient to clench his or her fist. Continuous clenching or pumping of the fist is not recommended because it will result in hemoconcentration, altering some test results. The tourniquet can be applied for only 1 minute; therefore, after the vein is located, the tourniquet should be removed while the site is being cleansed, and then reapplied immediately before the venipuncture.

Veins are located by sight and touch, referred to as palpation. The ability to feel a vein is much more important than the ability to see a vein. Palpation is performed by using the tip of the index finger to probe the antecubital area with a pushing rather than a stroking motion. Gloves should be worn when palpating veins to prevent contact with microorganisms such as methicillin-resistant *Staphylococcus aureus* (MRSA) and vancomycin-resistant enterococci (VRE).

Palpation is used to determine the size, depth, and direction of the vein to aid in directing the needle during insertion. The pressure applied by palpating locates deep veins and distinguishes veins, which feel like spongy cords, from rigid tendon cords. Veins must be differentiated from arteries, which produce a pulse; therefore, the thumb should not be used to palpate because it has a pulse beat. Select a vein that is easily palpated and large enough to support good blood flow.

Many patients have prominent veins in one arm and not in the other arm. Checking the patient's other arm should be the first thing done when a site is not easily located. Patients with veins that are difficult to locate often point out areas of previously successful phlebotomies. Palpation of these areas may prove beneficial and is also good for patient relations.

Other techniques to enhance the prominence of veins include gently tapping the antecubital area with the index finger, massaging the arm upward from the wrist to the elbow, briefly hanging the arm down, and applying heat to the site. Remember that the tourniquet should not remain tied for more than 1 minute at a time when performing these techniques.

If no palpable veins are found in the antecubital area, the wrist and hand should be examined. The tourniquet should be retied on the forearm. Because the veins in these areas are smaller, it may be necessary to change equipment and use a smaller needle with a syringe, a winged infusion set, or a smaller vacuum tube.

Veins in the legs and feet are sometimes used as venipuncture sites. They should be used only with physician approval. Leg veins are more susceptible to infection and the formation of clots (thrombi), particularly in patients with diabetes, cardiac problems, and coagulation disorders.

Veins that contain thrombi or that have been subjected to numerous venipunctures often feel hard (sclerosed) and should be avoided because they may be blocked (occluded) and the circulation may be impaired. Areas that appear blue or are cold may also have impaired circulation.

The presence of a hematoma indicates that blood has accumulated in the tissue surrounding a vein. Puncturing into a hematoma not only is painful for the patient but also results in the collection of old, hemolyzed blood from the hematoma rather than from circulating venous blood that is representative of the patient's current condition. If a vein containing a hematoma must be used, blood should be collected below the hematoma to ensure sampling of free-flowing blood. Drawing from areas containing excess tissue fluid (edema) is also not recommended because the sample will be contaminated with tissue fluid.

Extensively burned and scarred areas, including areas with tattoos, are more susceptible to infection; they also have decreased circulation and veins that are difficult to palpate.

Applying a tourniquet or drawing blood from an arm located on the same side of the body as a mastectomy can be harmful to the patient and produce erroneous test results. Removal of lymph nodes as part of the mastectomy procedure interferes with the flow of lymph fluid (lymphostasis) and increases the blood level of lymphocytes and waste products normally contained in the lymph fluid. Patients are in danger of developing lymphedema in the affected area. The protective functions of the lymphatic system are also lost, so that the area becomes more prone to infection. For these reasons, blood should be drawn from the other arm or possibly from the hand. In the case of a double mastectomy, the physician should be consulted as to an appropriate site. It may be possible to perform the tests from a fingerstick.

When a patient is receiving IV fluids, blood should be drawn from the other arm. If an arm containing an IV drip must be used for specimen collection, the site selected must be below the IV insertion point and preferably from a different vein. Whenever possible, areas near the site of a previous IV should be avoided for 24 to 48 hours. The IV drip should be turned off for at least 2 minutes and the first 5 mL of blood drawn must be discarded because it may be contaminated with IV fluid. When using a syringe, a new syringe must be used for the specimen collection. If a coagulation test is ordered, an additional 5 mL of blood (total of 10 mL) should be drawn before collecting the coagulation test specimen, because IV lines are frequently flushed with heparin. This additional blood can be used for other tests, if they have been ordered. When blood is collected from an arm containing an IV drip, it must be noted on the requisition form.

> **Technical Tip**
>
> Most mastectomy patients have been told never to have blood drawn from the affected side. Make sure they receive appropriate reassurance if an alternate site is not available.

> **Technical Tip**
>
> Inappropriate collection of blood from an arm containing an IV is a major cause of erroneous test results. Unless the specimen is highly contaminated, the error may not be detected.

CLEANSE THE SITE

> **Technical Tip**
>
> Patients are quick to complain about a painful venipuncture. The stinging sensation caused by undry alcohol is a frequent, yet easily avoided, cause of a complaint.

After the vein is located, release the tourniquet and cleanse the site using a 70 percent isopropyl alcohol wipe. Use a circular motion starting at the inside of the venipuncture site and work outward in widening concentric circles. For maximum bacteriostatic action to occur, the alcohol should be allowed to dry for 30 to 60 seconds on the patient's arm rather than being wiped off with a gauze pad. Performing a venipuncture before the alcohol has dried causes a stinging sensation for the patient and may hemolyze the specimen. Do not reintroduce contaminants by blowing on the site or fanning the area.

Blood cultures and arterial blood gases require that the site be cleansed with an antiseptic stronger than isopropyl alcohol. The most frequently used solutions are povidone-iodine or chlorhexidine gluconate, which is used for persons allergic to iodine.

Alcohol should not be used to cleanse the site prior to drawing a blood alcohol level. Thoroughly cleansing the site with soap and water ensures the least amount of interference, and some institutions find iodine to be acceptable.

EXAMINE AND ASSEMBLE PUNCTURE EQUIPMENT

While the alcohol is drying, make a final survey of the supplies at hand to be sure everything required for the procedure is present, and assemble the equipment.

Screw the stopper-puncturing end of the double-ended evacuated tube needle into the needle adapter. Do not remove the sterile cap from the other end of the needle. Insert the first tube to be collected into the needle adapter up to the designated mark. After the tube is pushed up to the mark, it may retract slightly when pressure is released. This is acceptable.

Immediately prior to the needle's entering the vein, remove the plastic cap and visually examine the point of the needle for any defects, such as a nonpointed or rough (barbed) end. Position the needle for entry into the vein with the bevel facing up.

Visual examination cannot detect all defective vacuum tubes; therefore, extra tubes should be at hand. It is not uncommon for the vacuum in a tube to be lost.

PERFORM THE VENIPUNCTURE

Reapply the tourniquet and confirm the puncture site. If necessary, cleanse the gloved palpating finger for additional vein palpation.

The needle holder or syringe is held securely in the dominant hand with the thumb on top and the other fingers below. After insertion is made, the fingers are braced against the patient's arm to provide stability while tubes are being moved in the adapter or the plunger of the syringe is being pulled back. Figure 3–4 provides additional illustration of the venipuncture procedure.

Use the thumb of the nondominant hand to anchor the selected vein while inserting the needle. Place the thumb 1 or 2 inches below the insertion site, and the four fingers on the back of the arm. Anchoring the vein above and below the site using the thumb and index finger is not an acceptable technique, because sudden patient movement could cause the index finger to be punctured. A vein that moves to the side is said to have "rolled." Patients often state that they have "rolling veins"; however, all veins will roll if they are not properly anchored. These patients are really saying that they have had blood drawn by practitioners who were not anchoring the veins well enough. As mentioned previously, the median cubital vein is the easiest to anchor and the basilic vein is the most difficult. In general, the closer a vein is to the surface, the more likely it is to roll.

When the vein is securely anchored, align the needle with the vein and insert it, bevel up, at an angle of 15 to 30 degrees depending on the depth of the vein (Figure 3–4A). It should be done in a smooth movement so the patient feels the stick only briefly. You will notice a feeling of lessening of resistance to the needle movement when the vein has been entered.

Technical Tip

Holding the adapter or syringe in the position used for injections prevents threading the needle into the vein or bracing the hand for exchange of tubes.

Figure 3–4

Performing the venipuncture. *A*, Needle insertion. *B*, Sample collection. *C*, Additional sample collection. *D*, Removal of needle, followed immediately by pressure to the puncture site.
(From Strasinger, SK, and Di Lorenzo, MA: Phlebotomy Workbook for the Multiskilled Healthcare Professional. FA Davis, Philadelphia, 1996, Figure 13–11, p. 210, with permission.)

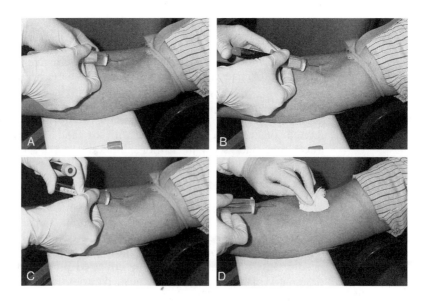

Once the vein has been entered, the hand anchoring the vein can be moved and used to push the evacuated tube completely into the adapter or to pull back on the syringe plunger (Figure 3–4B). Use the thumb to push the tube onto the back of the evacuated tube needle, while the index and middle fingers grasp the flared ends of the adapter. Blood should begin to flow into the tube, and the fist and tourniquet can be released, although if the procedure does not last more than 1 minute, the tourniquet can be left on until the last tube is filled. Some practitioners prefer to change hands at this point so that the dominant hand is free for performing the remaining tasks. Changing hands is usually better suited for use by experienced persons, because holding the needle steady in the patient's vein is often difficult for beginners.

The hand used to hold the needle assembly should remain braced on the patient's arm. This is of particular importance when vacuum tubes are being inserted or removed from the holder, because a certain amount of resistance is encountered and can cause the needle to be pushed through or pulled out of the vein. Tubes should be gently twisted on and off the puncturing needle (Figure 3–4C).

To prevent any chance of blood refluxing back into the needle, tubes should be held at a downward angle while they are being filled and have slight pressure applied to them. Be sure to follow the prescribed order of draw when multiple tubes are being collected, and allow the tubes to fill completely before removing them. Mixing of evacuated tubes should be done as soon as the tube is removed and before another tube is placed in the assembly. The few seconds required does not cause additional discomfort to the patient and ensures that the specimen will be acceptable.

When the last tube has been filled, it is removed from the assembly and mixed prior to completing the procedure. Failure to remove the evacuated tube before removing the needle causes blood to drip from the end of the needle, resulting in unnecessary contamination and possible damage to the patient's clothes.

REMOVE THE NEEDLE

Before removing the needle, remove the tourniquet by pulling on the free end, and tell the patient to relax his or her hand. Failure to remove the tourniquet before removing the needle may produce a bruise (hematoma).

Place folded sterile gauze over the venipuncture site, withdraw the needle, and apply pressure to the site as soon as the needle is withdrawn (Figure 3-4D). Do not apply pressure while the needle is still in the vein. To prevent blood from leaking into the surrounding tissue and producing a hematoma, pressure must be applied until the bleeding has stopped. The arm should be held in a raised, outstretched position. Bending the elbow to apply pressure allows blood to leak into the tissue more easily. A capable patient can be asked to apply the pressure, thereby freeing the blood collector to dispose of the used needle and label the specimen tubes. If this is not possible, the blood collector must apply the pressure and perform the other tasks after the bleeding has stopped.

DISPOSE OF THE CONTAMINATED NEEDLE

On completion of the venipuncture, the contaminated needle must be disposed of immediately in an acceptable sharps container conveniently located near the patient (Figure 3–5). As discussed in Unit 2, the method by which this is done depends on the type of disposal equipment selected by the institution. Under no circumstance should the needle be bent, cut, placed on a counter or bed, or manually recapped.

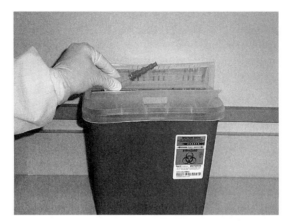

Figure 3-5

Needle disposal

LABEL THE TUBES

Tubes must be labeled at the time of specimen collection, before leaving the patient's room or accepting another outpatient requisition. Tubes are labeled by writing with a pen on the attached label or by applying a computer-generated label (Figure 3–6). Tubes should not be labeled before the specimen is collected, because this can result in confusion of specimens when more than one patient is having blood drawn or when a specimen cannot be collected. Preprinted labels should be verified before being attached to the specimen.

Information on the specimen label should include:

■ Patient's name and ID number
■ Date and time of collection
■ Collector's initials

Additional information may be present on computer-generated labels. The laboratory will reject incompletely and unlabeled tubes. Specimens for blood bank may require an additional label obtained from the patient's blood bank ID band.

Specimens requiring special handling, such as cooling or warming, are placed in the appropriate container when labeling is complete.

Figure 3-6

Labeling the tube
(From Strasinger, SK, and Di Lorenzo, MA: Phlebotomy Workbook for the Multi-skilled Healthcare Professional. FA Davis, Philadelphia, 1996, Figure 13-13, p. 211, with permission.)

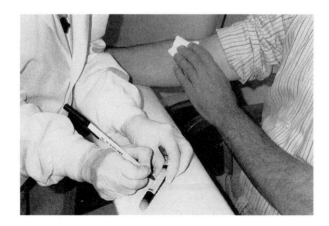

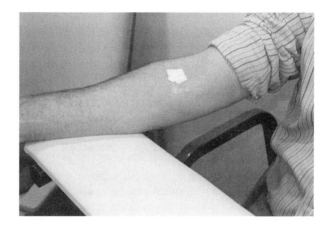

Figure 3–7

Patient's arm with bandage
(From Strasinger, SK, and Di Lorenzo, MA: Phlebotomy Workbook for the Multiskilled Healthcare Professional. FA Davis, Philadelphia, 1996, Figure 13–14, p. 212, with permission.)

BANDAGE THE PATIENT'S ARM

Technical Tip

The practice of quickly applying tape over the gauze without checking the puncture site frequently produces hematomas.

Bleeding at the venipuncture site should stop within 5 minutes. Before applying the bandage, the blood collector should examine the patient's arm to be sure the bleeding has stopped. For additional pressure, an adhesive bandage or tape is applied over a folded gauze square (Figure 3–7). The patient should be instructed to remove the bandage within 1 hour and to avoid using the arm to carry heavy objects during that period.

Patients receiving anticoagulant medications or large amounts of aspirin or patients with coagulation disorders may continue to bleed after pressure has been applied for 5 minutes. Continue to apply pressure until the bleeding has stopped.

In the case of an accidental arterial puncture, which usually can be detected by the appearance of unusually red blood that spurts into the tube, the blood collector, not the patient, should apply pressure to the site for 10 minutes. The fact that the specimen is arterial blood should be recorded on the requisition form.

Some patients are allergic to adhesive bandages, and it may be necessary to wrap gauze around the arm prior to applying the adhesive tape. Bandages are not recommended for children younger than 2 years old, because children may put bandages in their mouth.

DISPOSE OF USED SUPPLIES

Before leaving the patient's room, dispose of all contaminated supplies, such as alcohol, pads, and gauze in a biohazard container; remove gloves and dispose of them in the biohazard container; and wash your hands.

THANK THE PATIENT

Patients should be thanked for their cooperation in both inpatient and outpatient settings. Leave the patient's room in the condition in which you found it (bed and bedrails in the same position).

DELIVER SPECIMENS TO THE LABORATORY

Use designated containers for transport, and securely attach the requisitions with the specimen. Specimens must be delivered to the laboratory as soon as possible. Gently transport specimens in a vertical position to facilitate clotting and prevent hemolysis.

Blood specimens should be transported to the laboratory for processing as soon as possible. The stability of analytes varies greatly, as do the accepted methods of preservation. This is why rapid delivery to the laboratory or following laboratory prescribed specimen handling protocols is essential. Common protocols include separation of the plasma or serum from the cells (either manually or by gel), storage temperature, and protecting the specimen from exposure to light. Gel separation tubes must always be stored in an upright position.

The National Committee on Clinical Laboratory Standards (NCCLS) recommends centrifugation of clotted tubes and separation of the serum from the cells within 2 hours. Ideally, the specimen should reach the laboratory within 45 minutes and be centrifuged on arrival. Tests most frequently affected by improper processing include glucose, potassium, and coagulation tests. Glycolysis caused by the use of glucose in cellular metabolism causes falsely lower glucose values. Hemolysis and leakage of intracellular potassium into the serum or plasma falsely elevates potassium results. Coagulation factors are very labile, requiring the plasma to be refrigerated within ½ hour and tests performed within 4 hours. Appendix 3 summarizes the requirements of some routinely encountered analytes.

The venipuncture procedure is complete when the specimen is delivered to the laboratory in satisfactory condition and all appropriate paperwork has been completed. These procedures vary, depending on institutional protocol and the types of specimens collected.

SUMMARY OF VENIPUNCTURE TECHNIQUE USING AN EVACUATED TUBE SYSTEM

1. Obtain and examine the requisition form.
2. Greet the patient.
3. Identify the patient.
4. Reassure the patient and explain the procedure.
5. Prepare the patient.
6. Wash hands and put on gloves.
7. Select supplies and puncturing equipment.
8. Apply the tourniquet.
9. Select the venipuncture site.
10. Release the tourniquet.
11. Cleanse the site.
12. Survey and assemble equipment.
13. Reapply the tourniquet.
14. Confirm the venipuncture site.
15. Anchor the vein.
16. Insert the needle.
17. Push vacuum tube completely into adapter.
18. Mix the specimens, as they are collected.
19. Remove last tube from the holder.
20. Release the tourniquet.
21. Place sterile gauze over the needle.
22. Remove the needle and apply pressure.

23. Dispose of the needle.
24. Label the tubes.
25. Perform appropriate specimen handling.
26. Examine the patient's arm.
27. Bandage the patient's arm.
28. Dispose of used supplies.
29. Remove and dispose of gloves.
30. Wash hands.
31. Complete any required paperwork.
32. Thank the patient.
33. Deliver specimens to appropriate locations.

Evaluation of Venipuncture Technique Using an Evacuated Tube System

Rating System   2 = Satisfactory   1 = Needs Improvement   0 = Incorrect/Did Not Perform

_____ 1. Examines requisition form.
_____ 2. Greets patient and states procedure to be done.
_____ 3. Identifies the patient verbally.
_____ 4. Examines patient's ID band.
_____ 5. Compares requisition information with ID band.
_____ 6. Washes hands and puts on gloves.
_____ 7. Selects correct tubes and equipment for procedure.
_____ 8. Positions patient's arm.
_____ 9. Applies tourniquet.
_____ 10. Identifies vein by palpation.
_____ 11. Releases tourniquet.
_____ 12. Cleanses site and allows it to air dry.
_____ 13. Assembles equipment.
_____ 14. Reapplies tourniquet.
_____ 15. Does not touch puncture site with unclean finger.
_____ 16. Anchors vein below puncture site.
_____ 17. Smoothly enters vein at appropriate angle with bevel up.

_____ 18. Does not move needle when changing tubes.
_____ 19. Collects tubes in correct order.
_____ 20. Mixes anticoagulated tubes promptly.
_____ 21. Fills tubes completely.
_____ 22. Removes last tube collected from holder.
_____ 23. Releases tourniquet.
_____ 24. Covers puncture site with gauze.
_____ 25. Removes the needle smoothly and applies pressure.
_____ 26. Disposes of the needle in sharps container.
_____ 27. Labels tubes.
_____ 28. Examines puncture site.
_____ 29. Applies bandage.
_____ 30. Disposes of used supplies.
_____ 31. Removes gloves and washes hands.
_____ 32. Thanks patient.
_____ 33. Converses appropriately with patient during procedure.

Total points _____
Maximum points = 66
COMMENTS

U·N·I·T 4

Complications and
Additional Techniques

Learning Objectives

Upon completion of this unit, the reader will be able to:

- [ ] List the reasons why blood may not be immediately obtained from a venipuncture and the procedures to follow to obtain blood.

- [ ] List six causes of hematomas.

- [ ] Discuss the venipuncture errors that may produce hemolysis.

- [ ] Explain five causes of specimen contamination.

- [ ] Describe technical complications related to blood collection and the remedies for each situation.

- [ ] Discuss patient complications and an effective method to handle each situation.

- [ ] Describe the venipuncture procedure using a syringe, including equipment examination, technique for exchanging syringes, transfer of blood to evacuated tubes, and disposal of the equipment.

- [ ] Describe the venipuncture procedure using a butterfly, including technique involved and disposal of the equipment.

- [ ] Discuss the various types of central venous catheter devices and the requirements for blood collection.

- [ ] List five reasons for rejecting a specimen.

INTRODUCTION

Patient and procedural complications can occur with blood collection. Technical complications with the venipuncture procedure result in the inability to obtain blood, a rejected specimen, or discomfort to the patient. This unit identifies the complications that can be encountered and remedies for each. Additional techniques for obtaining blood in these special situations are also emphasized.

FAILURE TO OBTAIN BLOOD

The primary complication for the blood collector is the failure to obtain blood when the needle is inserted. Figure 4–1 illustrates possible causes of failure to obtain

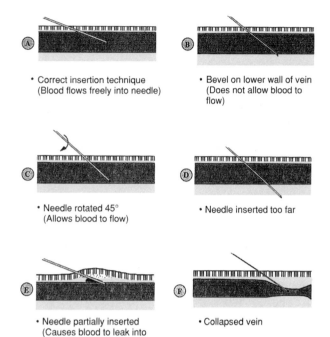

Figure 4-1

Possible reasons for failure to obtain blood (From Strasinger, SK, and Di Lorenzo, MA: Phlebotomy Workbook for the Multi-skilled Healthcare Professional. FA Davis, Philadelphia, 1996, Figure 14-3, p. 232, with permission.)

- Correct insertion technique (Blood flows freely into needle)
- Bevel on lower wall of vein (Does not allow blood to flow)
- Needle rotated 45° (Allows blood to flow)
- Needle inserted too far
- Needle partially inserted (Causes blood to leak into tissue)
- Collapsed vein

blood. Slightly moving or turning the needle may result in blood flow without having to repuncture the patient.

A frequent reason for the failure to obtain blood occurs when a vein is not well anchored prior to the puncture. The needle may slip to the side of the vein without actual penetration. Gently touching the area around the needle with a cleansed-gloved finger may determine the positions of the vein and the needle, and the needle can be slightly redirected. To avoid having to repuncture the patient, withdraw the needle until the bevel is just under the skin, reanchor the vein, and redirect the needle into the vein.

Blood flow may not occur when the angle of needle insertion is too steep (greater than 30 degrees) or when the tube adapter is not kept steady when tubes are advanced onto the needle. The needle may penetrate through the vein into the tissue. Gently pulling the needle back may produce blood flow.

If the needle angle is too shallow (less than 15 degrees), the needle may only partially enter the lumen of the vein, causing blood to leak into the tissues. Slowly advancing the needle into the vein may correct the problem.

Blood flow may also be prevented when the bevel of the needle is resting against the wall of the vein. Rotating the needle a quarter of a turn or pulling slightly back on the needle will allow blood to flow freely.

If the needle appears to be in the vein, a faulty evacuated tube (either by manufacturer error or accidental puncture when assembling the equipment) may be the problem and a new tube should be used. Remember to always have extra tubes within reach.

Using too large an evacuated tube or pulling back on the plunger of a syringe too quickly creates suction pressure that can cause a vein to collapse and stop blood flow. To remedy the situation, remove the tube, reapply the tourniquet if possible, and wait a few seconds for blood flow to return, and try using a smaller volume tube.

If this does not help, another puncture must be performed, possibly using a syringe or a butterfly.

It is important for blood collectors to know these techniques to avoid having the patient unnecessarily repunctured.

Movement of the needle should not include vigorous probing, because not only is this painful to the patient, but this also enlarges the puncture site and blood may leak into the tissues and form a hematoma.

When blood is not obtained from the initial venipuncture, the blood collector should select another site, either in the other arm or below the previous site, **and repeat the procedure using a new needle.** If the second puncture is not successful, the same person should not make another attempt. Possibly a phlebotomist from the clinical laboratory should attempt to collect the specimen.

HEMATOMAS

Hematomas are caused by the leakage of blood into the tissues around the venipuncture site. The skin discoloration and swelling that accompanies a hematoma is often a cause of anxiety and discomfort to the patient. Improper technique when removing the needle is a frequent cause of the appearance of a hematoma on the patient's arm. Errors in technique that cause blood to leak or to be forced into the surrounding tissue and produce hematomas include the following:

1. Failing to remove the tourniquet prior to removing the needle
2. Applying inadequate pressure to the site after removal of the needle
3. Excessive probing to obtain blood
4. Failing to insert the needle far enough into the vein
5. Inserting the needle through the vein
6. Bending the arm while applying pressure

Under normal conditions, the elasticity of the vein walls prevents the leakage of blood around the needle during venipuncture. A decrease in the elasticity of the vein walls in older patients causes them to be more prone to developing hematomas. If the area begins to form a hematoma while blood is being collected, immediately remove the tourniquet and needle and apply pressure to the site. Using small-bore needles and firmly anchoring the veins prior to needle insertion may prevent hematoma formation in these patients.

The compromised venipuncture site is unacceptable for blood collection until the hematoma is resolved. An alternate site should be chosen for venipuncture, or if none is available, the venipuncture must be performed below the hematoma. The goal of successful blood collection is not only to obtain the sample, but also to preserve the site for future venipunctures. It is critical to prevent hematoma formation.

Technical Tip

Specimens collected following vigorous probing are frequently hemolyzed and must be recollected.

HEMOLYZED SPECIMENS

Hemolysis is detected by the presence of pink or red plasma or serum. Rupture of the red blood cell membrane releases cellular contents into the serum or plasma and produces interference with many test results, which may require the specimen to be redrawn. Table 4–1 summarizes the major tests affected by hemolysis.

Table 4-1 Laboratory Tests Affected by Hemolysis

Seriously Affected	Noticeably Affected	Slightly Affected
Potassium (K)	Serum iron (Fe)	Phosphorus (P)
Lactic dehydrogenase (LD)	Alanine aminotransferase (ALT)	Total protein (TP)
Aspartate aminotransferase (AST)	Thyroxine (T4)	Albumin
Complete blood count (CBC)		Magnesium (Mg)
		Calcium (Ca)
		Acid phosphatase

Technical Tip

Hemolysis that is not evident to the naked eye can elevate critical potassium values.

Errors in performance of the venipuncture account for the majority of hemolyzed specimens and include:

1. Using a needle with too small a diameter (above 23 gauge)
2. Using a small needle with a large vacuum tube
3. Using an improperly attached needle on a syringe so that frothing occurs as the blood enters the syringe
4. Pulling the plunger of a syringe back too fast
5. Drawing blood from a site containing a hematoma
6. Vigorously mixing tubes
7. Forcing blood from a syringe into a vacuum tube
8. Failing to allow the blood to run down the side of an evacuated tube when using a syringe to fill it
9. Collecting specimens from IV lines when not recommended by the manufacturer
10. Applying the tourniquet too close to the puncture site or for too long

SPECIMEN CONTAMINATION

Specimen contamination affects the integrity of the specimen, causing invalid test results. The laboratory personnel may not know that contamination has occurred and consequently can report erroneous test results that adversely affect overall patient care. Incorrect blood collection techniques that cause contamination include:

1. Blood collected from edematous areas
2. Blood collected from veins with hematomas
3. Blood collected from arms containing an IV
4. Sites contaminated with alcohol
5. Anticoagulant carryover between tubes

TECHNICAL PROBLEMS

Rarely, the blood collector may encounter an evacuated tube that pops off the back of the adapter needle while blood is being collected. Readvancing the tube onto the needle in the adapter and holding it in this position until the tube is filled will remedy this situation.

Reflux of a tube anticoagulant can occur when there is blood backflow into a patient's vein from the collection tube. This can cause adverse reactions in patients. Keeping the patient's arm in a downward position, allowing the collection tubes to fill from the bottom up, eliminates this problem.

Partially filled collection tubes deliver the wrong ratio of blood to anticoagulant, resulting in an inadequate specimen for laboratory testing. Light-blue stopper tubes are the most affected because they contain liquid anticoagulant and the incorrect anticoagulant:blood ratio dilutes the plasma and causes erroneously prolonged coagulation results. The lavender stopper tube must be filled to avoid excess EDTA shrinking the red blood cells and affecting the hematocrit, red blood cell count, hemoglobin, red blood cell indices, and erythrocyte sedimentation rate (ESR) results. ESRs must be analyzed within 2 hours of the specimen collection. Completely filled green stopper tubes are critical for ionized calcium tests.

> *Technical Tip*
>
> **To ensure prevention of reflux, blood in the tubes should not come in contact with the stopper during collection.**

PATIENT COMPLICATIONS

> *Technical Tip*
>
> **Patients frequently mention previous adverse reactions. If these patients are sitting up, it may be wise to have them lie down prior to collection. It is not uncommon for patients with a history of fainting to faint again.**

Apprehensive patients may be prone to fainting (syncope). It is sometimes possible to detect such patients during vein palpation, because their skin may feel cold and damp. Keeping their minds off the procedure through conversation may be helpful. If a patient begins to faint during the procedure, remove the tourniquet and needle and apply pressure to the venipuncture site. Make certain a patient who is not in bed is supported and that the patient lowers his or her head. Applying cold compresses to the forehead and back of the neck helps revive the patient. Outpatients who have been fasting for prolonged periods should be given something sweet to drink and be required to remain in the area for 15 to 30 minutes. All incidents of syncope should be documented according to institutional policy.

It is rare for patients to develop seizures during venipuncture. If this happens, the needle and tourniquet should be removed, pressure applied to the site, and help summoned. Restrain the patient only to the extent that injury is prevented. Do not attempt to place anything in the patient's mouth. Any very deep puncture caused by sudden movement by the patient should be reported to the physician.

Patients who present with small, nonraised red hemorrhagic spots (called petechiae) may have prolonged bleeding following venipuncture. Petechiae can be an indication of a coagulation disorder, such as a low platelet count or abnormal platelet function.

Patient medications may interfere with the clinical interpretation of some test results. Acetaminophen (Tylenol) and erythromycin can increase serum aspartate aminotransferase (AST) and bilirubin levels. Intravenous injections of medications and dyes can also interfere with laboratory analysis. Blood creatinine, cortisol, and digoxin levels can be altered by the intravenous fluorescein used in angiography procedures. If the blood collector is aware of a recent dye injection or patient medication, it should be noted on the requisition. A complete list of drugs that can interfere with laboratory test results can be found in *Effects of Drugs on Clinical Laboratory Tests*, 4th Edition, by D. S. Young (AACC Press, Washington, DC, 1995).

Medications that are toxic to the liver can cause an increase in blood liver enzymes and abnormal coagulation tests. Elevated blood urea nitrogen (BUN) levels or imbalanced electrolytes may be seen in patients taking medications that impair renal function. Patients taking corticosteroids, estrogens, or diuretics can develop pancreatitis and would have elevated serum amylase and lipase levels. Hypobilirubinemia can be caused by a patient taking aspirin, because bilirubin is expelled from the plasma to the surrounding tissue cells. Communication between the blood collector and the laboratory staff concerning possible interfering medications will ensure quality patient test results.

USE OF SYRINGES

Except for a few minor differences, the procedure for drawing blood using a syringe is the same as when using an evacuated tube system. Blood is withdrawn from the vein by slowly pulling on the plunger of the syringe using the hand that is free after the anchored vein is entered. The advantage of using a syringe is that when the vein is entered, blood will appear in the hub of the needle and the plunger can then be pulled back at a speed that corresponds to the rate of blood flow into the syringe. Pulling the plunger back faster than the rate of blood flow may cause the walls of the vein to collapse (see Figure 4–1 *F*) and can cause hemolysis. It is important to anchor the hand holding the syringe firmly on the patient's arm so that the needle will not move when the plunger is pulled.

Ideally, the size of the syringe used should correspond to the amount of blood needed. It may be necessary to fill two or more smaller syringes when veins are small and may easily collapse. This will require assistance, because blood from the filled syringe must be transferred to the appropriate tubes while the second syringe is being filled. It is important that blood be added to anticoagulated tubes as soon as possible. Before exchanging syringes, gauze must be placed on the patient's arm under the needle because blood will leak from the hub of the needle during the exchange.

Technical Tip

In most circumstances, the use of small evacuated tubes instead of a syringe can prevent the need to change syringes.

As discussed in Unit 2, blood is transferred from the syringe to evacuated tubes, following the prescribed order of fill, by puncturing the rubber tube stopper using a one-handed technique and allowing the blood to flow slowly into the tube. After the tubes are filled, the syringe safety device is activated and the entire assembly is then discarded into a sharps container.

USE OF WINGED INFUSION SETS

All routine venipuncture procedures used with evacuated tubes and syringes also apply to blood collection using a winged infusion set (butterfly). This method is used for difficult venipuncture and is often less painful to patients. By folding the plastic needle attachments ("wings") upward while inserting the needle, the angle of insertion can be lowered to 10 to 15 degrees, thereby facilitating entry into small veins. Blood will appear in the tubing when the vein is entered. The needle can then be threaded securely into the vein and kept in place by holding the plastic wings against the patient's arm. It may be helpful to have a piece of tape available in case two hands are needed for the collection. Depending on the type of butterfly apparatus used, blood can be collected into an evacuated tube or a syringe. The tubing contains a small of amount of air that will cause underfilling of the first tube; therefore, a red stopper tube or discard tube should be collected before an anticoagulated tube to maintain the correct blood:anticoagulant ratio. To prevent hemolysis when using a small (23-gauge) needle, pediatric-size vacuum tubes should be used.

When disposing of the butterfly apparatus, use extreme care, because many accidental sticks result from unexpected movement of the tubing. Immediately activating the needle safety device and placing the needle into a sharps container and then allowing the tubing to fall into the container when the evacuated tube or

Figure 4-2

Venipuncture using a butterfly. *A*, Hand vein palpation. *B*, Cleansing the puncture site. *C*, Inserting the needle. *D*, Advancing an evacuated tube into the adapter. *E*, Blood flow through the butterfly apparatus. *F*, Removing the needle. *G*. Disposing of the butterfly apparatus. *H*, Patient's hand with pressure bandage.

(From Strasinger, SK, and Di Lorenzo, MA: Phlebotomy Workbook for the Multiskilled Healthcare Professional. FA Davis, Philadelphia, 1996, Figure 14–2, p. 231, with permission.)

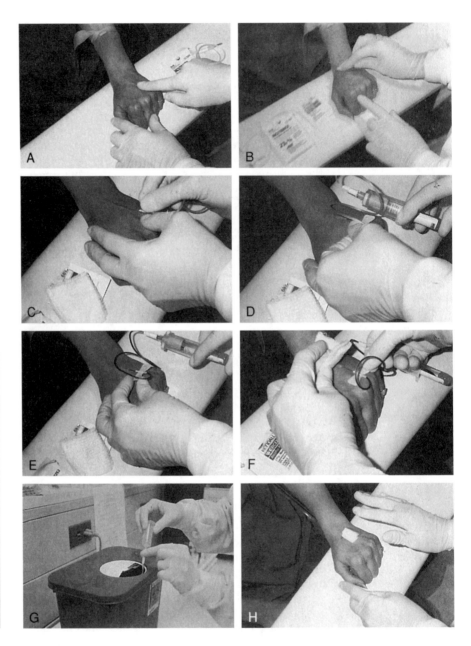

syringe is removed can prevent accidents. Always hold a butterfly apparatus by the wings, not by the tubing. Using an apparatus with automatic resheathing capability or activating a device on the needle set that advances a safety blunt before removing the needle from the vein also prevents accidental needle punctures. Do not push the apparatus manually into a full sharps container.

The venipuncture procedure using a butterfly is shown in Figure 4–2.

USE OF CENTRAL VENOUS CATHETERS

Blood specimens may be obtained from indwelling lines called central venous catheters (CVCs). There are numerous central venous access devices (CVADs), and this procedure requires that personnel have received special training in these collection procedures. Specific procedures must be followed for flushing the catheters with saline, and possibly heparin, when the blood collection is completed (see Appendix 4). Sterile technique procedures must be strictly adhered to when entering IV lines, because they provide a direct path for infectious organisms to enter the patient's bloodstream.

A central venous access device has a catheter with a tip lying in the superior vena cava that can be utilized for administration of fluids, drugs, blood products, nutritional solutions, and to obtain blood specimens. Four major categories of CVADs are used and include:

1. Nontunneled
2. Tunneled
3. Implanted portacaths
4. Peripherally inserted central catheters (PICCs)

The nontunneled CVAD is used for short-term dwell times and is inserted into the jugular, subclavian, or femoral vein by a physician in surgery or in a hospital room with local anesthetic. It can be a single, double, or triple lumen catheter. When using multilumen catheters, blood should be obtained from the most proximal lumen. The lumens not being used should be clamped when drawing blood, to avoid contamination of the blood sample. A dressing covers the tubing that extends above the skin, and flushes are necessary to maintain this CVC.

The tunneled CVAD is considered more permanent and is used for long-term dwell times, such as administration of chemotherapy. The Hickman and Groshong catheters are examples of this single or double lumen type of catheter. A surgeon performs a cut-down of the vein with local or IV sedation, using fluoroscopy to tunnel the catheter in subcutaneous tissue under the skin to the exit site and placing the catheter tip in the superior vena cava. Dressing changes and flushing with heparin or saline are required maintenance for this catheter.

The implanted portacath is a small chamber attached to an indwelling line that is also considered more permanent and is used for long-term access to the central venous system for a patient requiring frequent IVs or receiving chemotherapy. Using local or IV sedation, a surgeon implants the portacath in subcutaneous tissue under the skin with the catheter tip placed in the superior vena cava. The self-sealing septum of the device withstands 1000 to 2000 needle punctures; however, only noncoring needles called Huber needles can be used. The advantages of this CVAD is that there is no visible tubing and no site care is needed when it is not being used. It is flushed monthly with heparin or saline.

The peripherally inserted central catheter (PICC) is placed in the basilic or cephalic vein in the antecubital area of the arm, with the tip threaded to the superior vena cava. PICCs can be placed by IV team nurses or physicians and can be used for weeks to months. The advantages of a PICC is that has few risks and minimal discomfort for the patient.

Heparin or saline locks are winged infusion sets that can be left in a vein for up to 48 hours to provide a means for administering frequently required medications and for obtaining blood specimens. The devices must be flushed

Technical Tip

When blood is collected from a CVAD, blood should not be left in the syringe while extensive flushing of the CVAD is performed. Anticoagulation of the specimen also is important.

with heparin or saline periodically and after use to prevent blood clots from developing in the line.

When IV fluids are being administered through the CVC, the flow should be stopped for 5 minutes before collecting the sample. Syringes larger than 20 mL should not be used because the high negative pressure produced may collapse the catheter wall. At all times, the first 5 mL of blood must be discarded and a new syringe must be used to collect the sample. Drawing coagulation tests from a venous catheter is not recommended, but if this is necessary, the tests should be collected after 20 mL of blood have been discarded or used for other tests.

The order of tube fill may vary slightly to accommodate the amount of blood that must be drawn prior to a coagulation test. As with other procedures, blood cultures are always collected first. If blood cultures are ordered, the draw will satisfy the additional discard needed for coagulation tests. Therefore, the order of draw or fill is as follows:

1. First syringe – 5 mL discard
2. Second syringe – Blood cultures
3. Third syringe – Anticoagulated tubes (light-blue, lavender, green, and gray)
4. Clotted tubes (red and SST)

If blood cultures are not ordered, the coagulation tests (light-blue stopper tube) can be collected with a new syringe after the other specimens have been collected, using the order previously listed. The source of the specimen should be noted on the requisition form. Follow specific institutional protocol for obtaining blood from a CVAD.

CANNULAS AND FISTULAS

Patients receiving renal dialysis may have a permanent surgical fusion of an artery and a vein, called a fistula, or a temporary external connection called a cannula. Cannulas contain a special diaphragm from which blood can be collected by specially trained personnel.

Blood should not be collected from arms containing fistulas. Be sure to check for the presence of a cannula or fistula before applying a tourniquet to the arm, because this can compromise the patient.

CAUSES OF SPECIMEN REJECTION

Specimens brought to the laboratory may be rejected if conditions are present that would affect the validity of the test results.

Major reasons for specimen rejection are as follows:

1. Unlabeled or mislabeled specimens
2. Inadequate volume
3. Collection in the wrong tube
4. Hemolysis
5. Lipemia
6. Clotted blood in an anticoagulant tube
7. Improper handling during transport, such as not chilling the specimen
8. Specimens without a requisition form
9. Contaminated specimen containers

Venipuncture Situations *Exercise*

1. An unidentified patient in the emergency room requires a transfusion. What precautions must the blood collector take?

_____

_____

_____

2. The blood collector has a requisition to collect blood for a chemistry profile and a prothrombin time (PT). No blood is obtained from the left antecubital area. The blood collector then moves to the right antecubital area and obtains a full red stopper tube, but cannot fill the light-blue stopper tube. What should the blood collector do next?

_____

_____

_____

3. A patient has an IV drip running in the left forearm. From the following sites, indicate your first choice with a "1," your second choice with a "2," and an unacceptable site with an "X."
   a. _____ left wrist
   b. _____ left antecubital area
   c. _____ right antecubital area

4. The blood collector with a requisition for a PT, CBC, and glucose on a patient who is difficult to draw obtains 7 mL of blood using a syringe. Assuming the blood collector has a 2.7-mL light-blue stopper tube, a 2-mL lavender stopper tube, and a 3-mL red stopper tube, how should the blood be distributed?

_____

_____

_____

5. The blood collector is collecting blood for a PT, CBC, and a chemistry profile from an IV line:
   a. How many and what size syringes are needed and what is done with the blood collected in each?

_____

_____

_____

   b. What should the blood collector write on the requisition form?

_____

_____

_____

6. A blood collector needs to collect 20 mL of blood for serum chemistry tests and selects two 10-mL red stopper tubes. A successful puncture is performed; however, blood stops flowing when the first tube is only half full.
   a. Assuming the problem does not lie with the equipment, what is a possible reason for this?

_____

_____

b. State two methods the blood collector could use to collect the required amount of blood.

_____

_____

_____

7. When collecting a specimen from an elderly patient using routine evacuated tube equipment, the blood collector notices that the puncture site is beginning to swell.

   a. Why is this happening?

   _____

   b. What should the blood collector do?

   _____

   c. How can the specimen be collected?

   _____

8. While blood for a CBC is being collected, the patient develops syncope and the blood collector removes the needle and lowers the patient's head. Once the patient has recovered, the blood collector labels the lavender stopper tube, which fortunately contains enough blood, and delivers it to the clinical laboratory. Many results from this specimen are markedly lower than those from the patient's previous CBC.

   a. How could the quality of the specimen have caused this discrepancy?

   _____

   _____

   b. How could the venipuncture complication have contributed to this error?

   _____

   _____

   c. Could the blood collector have done anything differently? Explain your answer.

   _____

   _____

9. Patients in the cardiac care unit are exhibiting an unusual number of hematomas. Considering the condition and treatment of the patients in this unit, what is the most probable error being made by the blood collectors? Explain your answer.

   _____

   _____

   _____

10. The blood collector sends a properly labeled specimen with sufficient volume collected in a red stopper tube to the clinical laboratory for a potassium determination. Fifteen minutes later the chemistry supervisor calls and asks that the specimen be redrawn.

    a. Why did the chemistry section reject this specimen?

    _____

    b. What precautions should the blood collector take with the second specimen?

    _____

    _____

    _____

U·N·I·T 5

Special Venipuncture Collection

Learning Objectives

Upon completion of this unit, the reader will be able to:

- [ ] Explain the requirements for a 2-hour postprandial glucose test and a glucose tolerance test (GTT).

- [ ] Discuss diurnal variation of blood constituents and list three substances that would be affected.

- [ ] Differentiate between a trough and a peak level in therapeutic drug monitoring.

- [ ] Discuss the timing sequences for the collection of blood cultures, the reasons for selecting a particular timing sequence, and the number of specimens collected.

- [ ] Describe the procedure for collecting specimens for cold agglutinins.

- [ ] List eight tests for which specimens must be chilled immediately after collection.

- [ ] List five tests for which the results are affected by exposure of the specimen to light.

- [ ] Define chain of custody.

INTRODUCTION

Certain laboratory tests require the use of techniques that are not part of the routine venipuncture procedure. These nonroutine procedures may involve patient preparation, timing of specimen collection, venipuncture techniques, and specimen handling. The blood collector must know when these techniques are required, how to perform them, and how specimen integrity is affected when they are not performed.

FASTING AND TIMED SPECIMENS

Assessment of the patient preparation is necessary before blood collection for laboratory tests that require the patient to be fasting or in a basal state. It is the responsibility of the blood collector to verify that the patient has not had anything to eat or drink, except water, (fasting) and has refrained from strenuous exercise for 12 hours (basal state). Specimens for fasting blood sugar (FBS), triglycerides, and cardiac risk profiles are the most critically affected by nonfasting. If the patient has not fasted, it must be noted on the requisition form.

Blood collections are frequently requested for specific times, and the timing of specimen collection must be strictly followed for accurate test results. For example, collecting a specimen early could yield a falsely elevated result, whereas collecting the specimen late could yield a falsely normal result. Frequently encountered timed specimens are the 2-hour postprandial glucose, glucose tolerance test, therapeutic drug monitoring, and tests for substances that exhibit diurnal variation.

TWO-HOUR POSTPRANDIAL GLUCOSE

The 2-hour postprandial glucose test compares a patient's fasting glucose level with a glucose level 2 hours after eating a meal or ingesting a measured amount of glucose. It is used to evaluate diabetes mellitus. The blood collector must confirm that the patient has ingested a complete meal and collect the blood exactly 2 hours after the meal is ingested.

GLUCOSE TOLERANCE TEST

The glucose tolerance test (GTT) is a procedure performed for the diagnosis of diabetes mellitus (hyperglycemia) and for the evaluation of persons with symptoms associated with low blood glucose (hypoglycemia). The GTT compares glucose results on blood and urine collected at appropriate times. The specimen collection schedule for a 3- to 6-hour GTT is based on the time the patient finishes drinking the glucose solution. GTT procedures should be scheduled to begin between 0700 and 0900, because glucose levels exhibit a diurnal variation. A fasting glucose to determine whether the patient can safely be given a large amount of glucose is collected and tested prior to beginning the procedure. The patient drinks a standardized amount of flavored glucose within 5 minutes. The timing for the collection of the GTT specimens begins when the patient finishes drinking the glucose. Sample schedules are shown in Table 5–1.

Outpatients are given a copy of the schedule and instructed to continue fasting, to drink water as needed, and to return to the drawing station at the scheduled times. Patients are usually instructed to remain in the outpatient area.

Labels containing routinely required information and specimen order in the test

Technical Tip

When collecting GTT specimens, closely observe the patient for symptoms of hyperglycemia or hypoglycemia.

Table 5–1 Sample Glucose Tolerance Test Schedules

Test Procedure	3-hour Test	6-hour Test
Fasting blood and urine	0700	0700
Patient finishes glucose	0800	0800
½-hour specimen	0830	0830
1-hour specimen	0900	0900
2-hour specimen	1000	1000
3-hour specimen	1100	1100
4-hour specimen		1200
5-hour specimen		1300
6-hour specimen		1400

sequence, such as 1 hour, 2 hour, and so on, are placed on the specimens. Blood specimens that will not be tested until the end of the sequence should be collected in gray stopper tubes. Timing of specimen collection is critical, because test results are related to the scheduled times; any discrepancies should be noted on the requisition. Consistency of venipuncture or dermal puncture must also be maintained, because glucose values differ between the two types of blood.

Some patients may not be able to tolerate the glucose solution, and if vomiting occurs, the time of the vomiting must be reported and the physician must be contacted for a decision concerning whether to continue the test. Vomiting early in the procedure is considered most critical and usually requires the procedure to be rescheduled.

DIURNAL VARIATION

In addition to glucose, other substances such as cortisol, hormones, and serum iron also exhibit diurnal variation, and the levels of these substances fluctuate noticeably throughout the day. Certain variations can be substantial. For example, plasma cortisol levels collected between 0800 and 1000 will be twice as high as levels collected at 1600, and serum iron levels collected in the morning are one-third higher than those collected in the evening. Specimens must be collected at the specified time or the physician should be notified and the test rescheduled for the next day.

THERAPEUTIC DRUG MONITORING

Technical Tip

Depending on the half-life of the medication, the timing of peak levels in therapeutic drug monitoring can be critical.

The blood levels of some therapeutic drugs are monitored to ensure safety and medication effectiveness. Frequently monitored drugs include digoxin, gentamicin, tobramycin, vancomycin, and theophylline. The trough level is collected right before the next dose of medication is scheduled. The peak level is collected after medication administration at the time when the manufacturer specifies that the blood level should be at the highest point. The time of the peak level varies with the medication and the method of administration (IV, intramuscular, or oral). To ensure correct documentation of peak and trough levels, requisitions and specimen tube labels should include the time and method of administration of the last dose given, as well as the time that the specimen is collected.

BLOOD CULTURES

Blood cultures are requested to detect septicemia in febrile patients. Specimens are usually collected in sets of two, drawn either 1 hour apart or just before the patient's temperature spikes. If antibiotics are to be started immediately, the sets are drawn at the same time from different sites. Specimens collected from multiple sites at the same time serve as controls for possible contamination and must be labeled as to the collection site, such as right arm antecubital vein, and their number in the series (#1, #2, #3). A known skin contaminant must be cultured from at least two of the sites for it to be considered a possible pathogen.

Blood for the culture may be drawn directly into bottles containing culture media, transferred to the bottles from a syringe, or drawn into sterile tubes containing anticoagulant and transferred to culture media in the laboratory. An anticoagulant must be present in the tube or the medium to prevent microorganisms from being trapped within a clot, where they might be undetected. Blood culture bottles must be mixed after the blood is added. The anticoagulant sodium

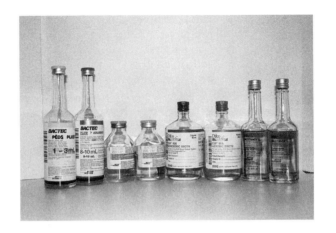

Figure 5-1

Types of blood culture collection systems

(From Strasinger, SK, and Di Lorenzo, MS: Skills for the Patient Care Technician. FA Davis, Philadelphia, 1999, Figure 8-1, p. 189, with permission).

polyanetholesulfonate (SPS) is used for blood cultures because it does not inhibit bacterial growth and may enhance it by inhibiting the action of phagocytes, complement, and some antibiotics. Other anticoagulants should not be used. Some blood culture collection systems have antimicrobial removal devices (ARDs) containing a resin that inactivates antibiotics. As shown in Figure 5–1, a variety of blood culture collection systems are available.

Strict adherence to aseptic technique during specimen collection is essential to ensure that a positive blood culture is not caused by external contamination. Cleansing of the venipuncture site begins by vigorous scrubbing of the site with alcohol for 60 seconds. The alcohol is followed by povidone-iodine applied by starting in the center and progressing outward in concentric circles. The iodine must be allowed to dry for 1 minute. If the site must be touched after cleansing, the gloved palpating finger must be cleaned in the same manner. The tops of the collection containers are also cleaned with iodine or alcohol and allowed to dry prior to inoculation. To prevent irritation of the arm, remove the iodine with alcohol when the procedure is complete.

Two specimens are routinely collected for each blood culture set, one to be incubated aerobically and the other to be incubated anaerobically. When a syringe is used, the anaerobic bottle should be inoculated first to prevent possible exposure to air.

A 1:10 ratio of blood to culture medium is critical, because the number of microorganisms present in the blood is often small. Pediatric collection containers are available.

> **Technical Tip**
>
> The National Committee on Clinical Laboratory Standards (NCCLS) recommends removing the dried alcohol or iodine from the blood culture stopper with clean gauze prior to inoculation.

SPECIAL SPECIMEN HANDLING PROCEDURES

Instructions for the collection, transportation, and storage of all laboratory specimens are available from the laboratory and should be strictly followed to maintain specimen integrity. Some tests require that the specimen be kept warm, chilled, frozen, or protected from light.

COLD AGGLUTININS

Cold agglutinins are autoantibodies produced by persons infected with *Mycoplasma pneumoniae*. The autoantibodies react with red blood cells at temperatures below body temperature. Because the cold agglutinins in the serum attach to red blood cells (RBCs) when the blood cools to below body temperature, the specimen must be kept warm until the serum can be separated from the cells. Specimens are collected in tubes that have been warmed in an incubator at 37°C for 30 minutes and that contain no additives or gels that could interfere with the test. The warmed tube is carried to the patient's room in the blood collector's tightly closed fist or a prewarmed container. The specimen is collected as quickly as possible and immediately delivered to the laboratory in the same manner. Failure to keep a specimen warm prior to serum separation produces falsely decreased test results.

CHILLED SPECIMENS

Technical Tip

Bilirubin is rapidly destroyed in specimens exposed to light.

Specimens for arterial blood gases, ammonia, lactic acid, pyruvate, gastrin, adrenocorticotropic hormone (ACTH), parathyroid hormone, and some coagulation studies must be chilled immediately after collection to prevent deterioration. For adequate chilling, the specimen must be placed in a mixture of crushed ice and water at the bedside. Placing a specimen in or on ice cubes is not acceptable, because uniform chilling will not occur. It is important that these specimens be immediately delivered to the laboratory for processing.

SPECIMENS SENSITIVE TO LIGHT

Exposure to light will decrease the concentration of bilirubin, beta-carotene, vitamins A and B_6, and porphyrins. Wrapping the tubes in aluminum foil can protect specimens.

LEGAL SPECIMENS

Technical Tip

Technical errors and failure to follow chain of custody protocol are primary targets of the defense in legal proceedings.

The chain of custody must be followed exactly when drawing specimens for test results that may be used as evidence in legal proceedings. Special forms are provided for the documentation of specimen handling, and special containers and seals may be required. Documentation must include the date, time, and identification of each person handling the specimen. Specimens should not be left sitting on a counter unattended. Patient identification and specimen collection should take place in the presence of a witness, often a law enforcement officer. Identification requires specific documents and may require photographs, fingerprints, or heel prints. The tests requested most frequently are alcohol and drug levels and DNA analysis.

When collecting blood alcohol levels, the site should be cleansed with soap and water or a nonalcoholic antiseptic solution. To prevent the escape of the volatile alcohol into the atmosphere, tubes should be filled completely and not uncapped prior to delivery to the laboratory. Blood alcohol levels are frequently collected in gray stopper tubes; however, laboratory protocol should be strictly followed.

Special Venipuncture Collection *Exercise*

1. An outpatient comes to the collection station at 1300 with a requisition for a cardiac risk profile. What should the blood collector ask the patient before collecting the specimen?

_____

_____

_____

2. Requisitions are received requesting that specimens for hemoglobin and hematocrit be collected at 0800, 1200, 1600, and 2000 from a patient on a medical-surgical unit. Is there a reason for these requests and, if so, what is it?

_____

_____

_____

3. An outpatient comes to the collection area with a requisition for a FBS and 2-hour pp glucose. What procedure should be followed?

_____

_____

_____

4. A patient receiving a 3-hour GTT vomits 20 minutes before the 3-hour specimen is scheduled. What should the blood collector do?

_____

_____

_____

5. A cortisol level is ordered on a patient scheduled to go to physical therapy at 0900. How would this patient be scheduled? Explain your answer.

_____

_____

_____

6. Would it be unusual to receive requests to collect theophylline levels at 0800 and again at 1200? Explain your answer.

_____

_____

_____

7. A request to draw three blood cultures within 30 minutes from a patient in the emergency room was made by the health-care provider. Is this a reasonable request? Why or why not?

_____

_____

_____

8. Two blood culture sets were collected in yellow stopper tubes and one in a lavender stopper tube and each transferred to bottles containing culture media. A known skin contaminant is cultured from two specimens.

   a. What errors in technique does this scenario indicate?

   _____

   _____

   _____

   b. Why was one culture negative?

   _____

   _____

   _____

9. Specimens for a stat ammonia level, a cold agglutinin test, and a CBC were collected, each from a different patient on opposite ends of the unit. The three specimens are sent to the laboratory in the pneumatic tube system. How will the quality of these test results be affected and why?

_____

_____

_____

10. As the attorney for a defendant charged with having a blood alcohol level above the legal limit, you are questioning the health-care professional who collected the specimen.

   a. State three questions you would ask the blood collector to try to discredit the test result.

   _____

   _____

   _____

   b. How should a competent health-care professional answer these questions?

   _____

   _____

   _____

Dermal Puncture

Upon completion of this unit, the reader will be able to:

☐ State the reasons for performing a dermal puncture.

☐ Describe the composition of capillary blood.

☐ Discuss the types of skin puncture devices available.

☐ Describe the four types of microspecimen containers.

☐ Discuss the purpose and methodology for puncture site warming.

☐ Identify the acceptable site for performing heel and finger punctures.

☐ List four unacceptable areas for performing heel puncture.

☐ State the complications produced by the presence of alcohol at the puncture site.

☐ State the correct positioning of the lancet for dermal puncture.

☐ Name the major cause of microspecimen contamination.

☐ State the order of collection for dermal puncture specimens.

☐ Describe the correct labeling of microspecimens.

INTRODUCTION

Advances in laboratory instrumentation and the popularity of point-of-care testing have made it possible to perform a majority of laboratory tests on microsamples of blood obtained by dermal puncture on both pediatric and adult patients. This unit presents the required equipment and correct procedure necessary for dermal punctures to provide a quality specimen.

Dermal puncture is the method of choice for collecting blood from infants and children younger than 2 years of age. Locating superficial veins large enough to accept even a small-gauge needle is difficult in these patients, and veins that are available may need to be reserved for IV therapy. Use of deep veins, such as the femoral vein, can be dangerous and may cause complications including cardiac arrest, venous thrombosis, hemorrhage, damage to surrounding tissue and organs, infection, reflex arteriospasm (which can possibly result in gangrene), and injury caused by restraining the child. Drawing excessive amounts of blood from premature and small infants can rapidly cause anemia, because a 2-lb infant may have a total blood volume of only 150 mL.

In adults, dermal puncture may be required for a variety of reasons, including:

1. Burned or scarred patients
2. Patients receiving chemotherapy who require frequent tests and whose veins must be reserved for therapy
3. Patients with thrombotic tendencies
4. Geriatric or other patients with very fragile veins
5. Patients with inaccessible veins
6. Home glucose monitoring and point-of-care testing

It may not be possible to obtain a satisfactory specimen by dermal puncture from patients who are severely dehydrated or who have poor peripheral circulation. Certain tests may not be collected by dermal puncture because of the larger amount of blood required; these include some coagulation studies, erythrocyte sedimentation rates, and blood cultures.

IMPORTANCE OF CORRECT COLLECTION

When collecting specimens for neonatal bilirubin tests, turn off the bili light during collection.

Correct collection techniques are critical because of the smaller amount of blood that is collected and the higher possibility of specimen contamination, microclots, and hemolysis. Hemolysis is more frequently seen in specimens collected by dermal puncture than it is in those collected by venipuncture. Excessive squeezing of the puncture site to obtain enough blood is often the cause of hemolysis. The presence of hemolysis may not be detected in specimens containing bilirubin, but it interferes not only with the tests routinely affected by hemolysis, but also with the frequently requested neonatal bilirubin determination.

COMPOSITION OF CAPILLARY BLOOD

Blood collected by dermal puncture comes from the capillaries, arterioles, and venules and may also contain small amounts of tissue fluid. Because of arterial pressure, the composition of this blood more closely resembles arterial blood than venous blood. With the exception of arterial blood gases, few chemical differences exist between arterial and venous blood. The concentration of glucose is higher in blood obtained by dermal puncture than it is in blood obtained by venipuncture, and the concentrations of potassium, total protein, and calcium are lower. Alternating between dermal puncture and venipuncture should not be done when results are to be compared. Note on the requisition form if the specimen is from a dermal puncture.

DERMAL PUNCTURE EQUIPMENT

Dermal puncture supplies include lancets or automatic puncture devices, micro-sample collection containers, 70 percent isopropyl alcohol pads, sterile gauze pads, bandages, an acceptable sharps container, heel warmers, marking pen, glass slides,

Figure 6-1

Skin puncture devices
(From Strasinger, SK, and Di Lorenzo, MS: Skills for the Patient Care Technician. FA Davis, Philadelphia, 1999, Figure 9–1, p. 200, with permission.)

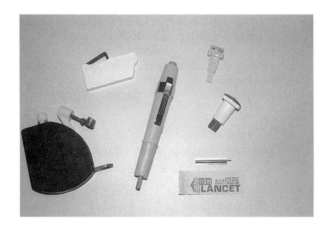

and gloves. With the exception of puncture devices, collection containers, heel warmers, and glass slides, the same equipment is also used for venipuncture.

SKIN PUNCTURE DEVICES

A variety of skin puncture devices are available, ranging from simple manual lancets to laser lancets (Figure 6–1). Many of the devices have retractable blades, which are recommended to avoid possible exposure to blood-borne pathogens. To prevent contact with bone, the depth of the puncture produced by a device is critical. Manufacturers provide separate devices designed for heelsticks and fingersticks on infants and children and fingersticks on adults. The length of manual lancets and spring release mechanisms or platforms controls the puncture depth with automatic devices. Punctures should never be performed using a surgical blade.

To produce adequate blood flow, the depth of the puncture is actually less important than the width of the puncture. As shown in Figure 6–2, the major vascular area of the skin is located at the dermal-subcutaneous juncture. The depth of this juncture can range from 0.35 mm in neonates to 2.4 mm in a large adult. Designated puncture devices easily reach it. Therefore, the number of severed capillaries depends on the width of the incision. Sufficient blood flow should be obtained from incision widths no larger than 2.5 mm.

As illustrated in the following examples, lancets are available in varying depths and widths. BD Vacutainer Safety Flow Lancets (Becton Dickinson, Franklin Lakes, NJ) are available in yellow (2.2 mm depth, 1.0 mm width) for heelsticks, blue (1.9 mm depth, 1.0 mm width) for microcollection tubes, green (1.4 mm depth, 1.0 mm depth) for point-of-care testing, and pink (1.4 mm depth, 0.5 mm width)

Figure 6-2

Vascular area of the skin
(Adapted from product literature, Becton Dickinson, Franklin Lakes, NJ.)

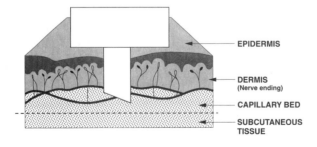

EPIDERMIS

DERMIS
(Nerve ending)

CAPILLARY BED

SUBCUTANEOUS TISSUE

**Orange Genie
Needle Lancet**
Designed for
glucose testing

**Pink Genie
Lancet**
Designed to fill a
hematocrit tube and
a drop of blood for
glucose testing

**Green Genie
Lancet**
Designed to fill a BD™
microcollection tube

**Blue Genie
Lancet**
Designed to fill a BD™
microcollection tube

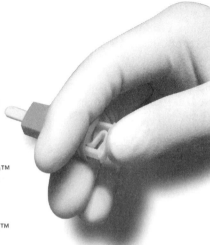

Figure 6-3

Genie safety lancet

(Courtesy of Becton Dickinson, Franklin Lakes, NJ.)

for glucose monitoring. Also available from BD is the Genie Safety Lancet offering one-step blade activation in varying depths. The orange Genie needle lancet (2.25 mm) provides a single blood drop used for glucose monitoring, the pink Genie lancet (1.0 mm depth, 1.5 mm width) is used for low blood flow, the green Genie lancet (1.5 mm depth, 1.5 mm width) for medium blood flow, and the blue Genie lancet (2.0 mm depth, 1.5 mm width) for medium to high blood flow (Figure 6–3). The BD Quikheel Lancet has a permanent retractable blade that minimizes possible injury or reuse. The color-coded heelstick lancets are made specifically for premature infants, newborns, and babies. The pink lancet has a depth of 0.85 mm and a width of 1.75 mm for premature infants, and the green lancet has a depth of 1.0 mm and a width of 2.50 mm (Figure 6–4).

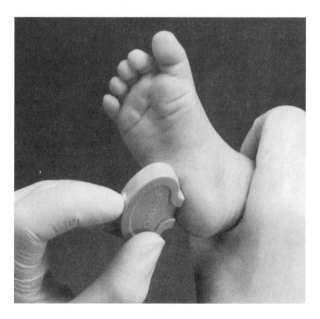

Figure 6-4

Quikheel lancet

(Courtesy of Becton Dickinson, Franklin Lakes, NJ.)

International Technidyne Corporation (Edison, NJ) provides a range of color-coded fully automated, single-use, retractable, disposable devices in varying depths. Tenderfoot and Tenderlett devices are designed for heel and finger punctures, respectively. Models are available ranging from the Tenderfoot for preemies to the Tenderlett for adults.

The Autolet systems (Ulster Scientific, Inc., New Paltz, NY) use disposable platforms to control the depth of the spring-activated puncture devices. The color-coded platforms are available in three depths ranging from 1.8 mm to 3.0 mm deep.

Laser systems are on the market for adults and children 5 years of age and older. The laser device eliminates the risks of accidental punctures or the need for sharps containers. The laser penetrates the skin 1 to 2 mm, creating a smaller wound, and up to 100 µL of blood can be collected.

MICROSPECIMEN CONTAINERS

Figure 6–5 illustrates some of the major specimen containers available for collection of microsamples, including capillary tubes, micropipets, microcollection tubes, and micropipets with dilution systems. Some containers are designated for a specific test, and others serve multiple purposes.

Capillary Tubes

Capillary tubes, frequently referred to as microhematocrit tubes, are small tubes used to collect approximately 50 to 75 mL of blood for the primary purpose of performing a microhematocrit. The tubes are designed to fit into a hematocrit centrifuge and its corresponding hematocrit reader. Tubes are available plain or coated with ammonium heparin and are color-coded with a red band for heparinized tubes and a blue band for plain tubes. Heparinized tubes should be used for hematocrits collected by dermal puncture, and plain tubes are used when the test is being performed on previously anticoagulated blood. When sufficient blood has been collected, the end of the capillary tube that has not been used to collect the specimen is closed by embedding it in a clay sealant designated for use with the tubes. Tubes protected by plastic sleeves and self-sealing tubes are available to prevent breakage when collecting specimens and sealing the microcapillary tubes.

Figure 6-5

Microspecimen containers

(From Strasinger, SK, and Di Lorenzo, MS: Skills for the Patient Care Technician. FA Davis, Philadelphia, 1999, Figure 9–3, p. 201, with permission.)

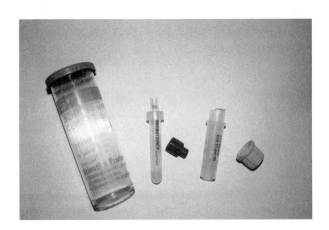

Micropipets

Larger capillary tubes, called Caraway or Natelson pipets, are used when tests other than a microhematocrit are requested. The pipets have a tapered end for specimen collection and fill by capillary action. Pipet lengths vary from 75 mm for Caraway pipets to 220 to 420 mL in Natelson pipets. Pipets are available plain or with ammonium heparin and are color-coded, respectively, with blue or red bands. After collection of the sample, the nontapered ends are sealed with specifically matched soft plastic caps or clay sealant.

Microcollection Tubes

Plastic collection tubes such as the Microtainer (Becton Dickinson, Franklin Lakes, NJ) provide a larger collection volume and present no danger from broken glass. A variety of anticoagulants and additives, including separator gel, are available, and the tubes are color-coded in the same way as evacuated tubes. Microtainer tubes have a microguard closure designed to reduce the risk of blood spatter and blood leakage. The microguard closure is removed by twisting and lifting. Tubes have a wide diameter, textured interior, and a blood collection scoop to enhance blood flow into the tube. After completion of the collection of blood, the cap is placed on the container, and anticoagulated tubes are gently inverted 10 times to ensure complete mixing. Tubes have markings to indicate minimum and maximum collection amounts to prevent underfilling or overfilling that could cause erroneous results. Separation of serum or plasma is achieved by centrifugation in specifically designed centrifuges.

Micropipet and Dilution System

The Unopette system (Becton Dickinson, Franklin Lakes, NJ) is designed for tests that can be performed on diluted whole blood, primarily hematology tests. The system consists of a sealed plastic reservoir containing a measured amount of diluent, a calibrated capillary pipet, and a plastic pipet shield. The amount and type of diluent and the size of the capillary pipet correspond to the specific test to be run. Pipets are designed to collect only the amount of blood for which they are calibrated.

DERMAL PUNCTURE PROCEDURE

Many of the procedures associated with venipuncture also apply to dermal puncture; therefore, major emphasis in this unit is on the techniques and complications that are unique to dermal puncture.

PREPUNCTURE PREPARATION

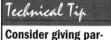

Technical Tip

Consider giving parents the option to stay with a child or leave the room.

The requisition provides the information as to the age of the patient and the test requested. This determines which of the variety of puncture devices and collection containers should be used for the dermal puncture. Patient identification may require confirmation from a parent or guardian.

When a specimen is collected by dermal puncture, it must be noted on the requisition form, because the concentration of some substances differs in venous and capillary blood.

PATIENT PREPARATION

For optimum blood flow, the area to be punctured should be warm. This is primarily a concern for patients with very cold or cyanotic fingers, for heelsticks to collect multiple samples, and for the collection of capillary blood gases. Warming dilates the blood vessels and increases arterial blood flow. Warming is performed by moistening a towel with warm water (40°C) or by activating a commercial heel warmer and covering the site for 3 to 5 minutes.

SITE SELECTION

The choice of a puncture area is based on the age and size of the patient. Select puncture sites that provide sufficient distance between the skin and the bone to avoid accidental contact with the bone that may cause infection (osteomyelitis). The primary sites are the heel, big toe, and the distal segments of the third and fourth fingers. Performing dermal punctures on earlobes is usually not recommended.

Areas selected for dermal puncture should not be callused, scarred, bruised, edematous, or infected. Punctures should never be made through previous puncture sites, because this can easily introduce microorganisms into the puncture and allow them to reach the bone.

Heel Puncture Sites

The heel is the most common site for dermal punctures on infants younger than 1 year of age, because it contains more tissue than the fingers and has not yet become callused from walking. Acceptable areas for heel puncture are shown in Figure 6–6 and are described as the medial and lateral areas of the bottom (plantar) surface of the heel. These areas can be determined by drawing imaginary lines extending back from the middle of the large toe and from between the fourth and fifth toes. It is in these areas that the distance between the skin and the heel bone (calcaneus) is greatest. Notice the short distance between the back (posterior curvature) of the heel and the calcaneus. This is the reason that this area is never acceptable for heel puncture.

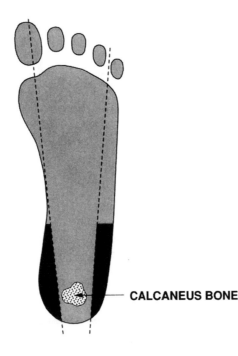

Figure 6-6

Acceptable heel puncture sites
(From Strasinger, SK, and Di Lorenzo, MA: Phlebotomy Workbook for the Multi-skilled Healthcare Professional. FA Davis, Philadelphia, 1996, Figure 16-5, p. 268, with permission.)

CALCANEUS BONE

Punctures should not be performed in other areas of the foot, and particularly not in the arch, where they may cause damage to nerves and tendons. In larger infants, the plantar surface of the large toes may be used. Physicians may specify the use of the big toe.

Finger Puncture Sites

Finger punctures are performed on adults and children older than 1 year of age. Fingers of infants younger than 1 year old may not contain enough tissue to prevent contact with the bone.

The fleshy areas located near the center of the third and fourth fingers on the palmar side are the sites of choice for finger puncture (Figure 6–7). Because the tip and sides of the finger contain only about half the tissue mass of the central area, the possibility of bone injury is increased in these areas. Problems associated with the use of other fingers include possible calluses on the thumb, increased nerve endings in the index finger, and decreased tissue in the fifth finger.

Summary of Dermal Puncture Site Selection

1. Use the medial and lateral areas of the plantar surface of the heel.
2. Use the central fleshy area of the third or fourth fingers.
3. Use the big toe in infants.
4. Do not use the back of the heel.
5. Do not use the arch of the foot.
6. Do not puncture through old sites.
7. Do not use areas with visible damage.

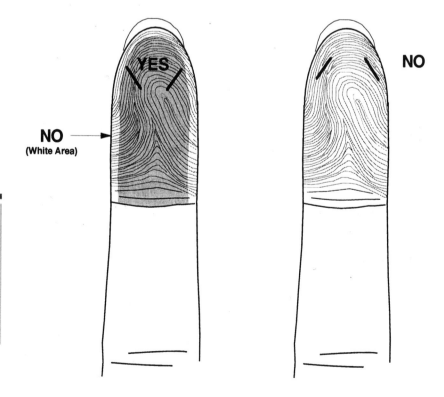

Figure 6-7

Acceptable finger puncture sites and correct puncture angle (From Strasinger, SK, and Di Lorenzo, MA: Phlebotomy Workbook for the Multi-skilled Healthcare Professional. FA Davis, Philadelphia, 1996, Figure 16-6, p. 269, with permission.)

CLEANSING THE SITE

The selected site is cleansed with 70 percent isopropyl alcohol using a circular motion. The alcohol should be allowed to dry on the skin for antiseptic action, and the residue removed with sterile gauze to prevent possible interference with test results. Failure to allow the alcohol to dry will:

1. Cause a stinging sensation for the patient.
2. Contaminate the specimen.
3. Hemolyze red blood cells (RBCs).
4. Prevent formation of a rounded blood drop because blood will mix with the alcohol and run down the finger.

Use of povidone-iodine is not recommended for dermal punctures because specimen contamination may elevate some test results, including bilirubin, phosphorus, uric acid, and potassium.

PERFORMING THE PUNCTURE

While the puncture is performed, the heel or finger should be well supported and held firmly, without squeezing the puncture area. Massaging the area before the puncture may increase blood flow to the area. The heel is held between the thumb and index finger of the nondominant hand (Figure 6–8). The finger is held between

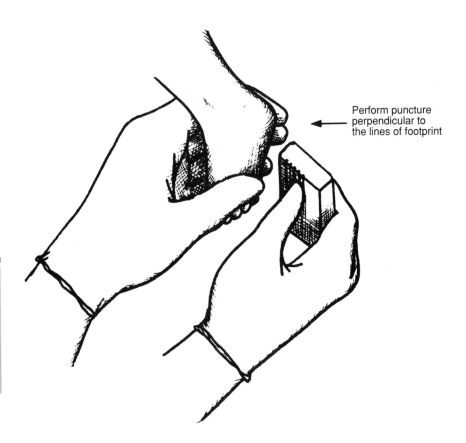

Perform puncture perpendicular to the lines of footprint

Figure 6–8

Correct position for heel puncture
(From Strasinger, SK, and Di Lorenzo, MA: Phlebotomy Workbook for the Multi-skilled Healthcare Professional. FA Davis, Philadelphia, 1996, Figure 16–7, p. 270, with permission.)

the thumb and index finger with the palmar surface facing up and the finger pointing downward to increase blood flow.

Punctures performed with a manual lancet should be made with one continuous motion, and automatic devices should be placed firmly on the puncture site. Do not indent the skin when placing the lancet on the puncture site. The blade of the lancet should be aligned to cut across (perpendicular to) the grooves of the finger or heel print (see Figure 6–7). This prevents the blood from running into the grooves, which prevents the formation of a rounded drop of blood. Depress the lancet and hold for a moment, then release. Pressure must be maintained, because the elasticity of the skin naturally inhibits penetration of the blade. Removal of the lancet before the puncture is complete will yield a low blood flow.

After completing the puncture, the lancet should be placed in an appropriate sharps container. A new puncture device must be used if an additional puncture is required.

> ### Technical Tip
>
> Failure to place puncture devices firmly on the skin is the primary cause of insufficient blood flow. One firm puncture is less painful for the patient than two "mini" punctures.

SPECIMEN COLLECTION

> ### Technical Tip
>
> Applying pressure about ½ inch away from the puncture site frequently produces better blood flow than pressure very close to the site.

Before beginning the collection, wipe away the first drop of blood with sterile gauze. This will prevent contamination of the specimen with residual alcohol and tissue fluid released during the puncture. When collecting microspecimens, even a minute amount of contamination can severely affect the sample quality. Therefore, blood should be flowing freely from the puncture site as a result of firm pressure and should not be obtained by milking or strenuous massaging of the surrounding tissue, which will release tissue fluid. The most satisfactory blood flow is obtained by alternately applying and releasing pressure to the area. Tightly squeezing the area with no relaxation cuts off blood flow to the puncture site.

Because collection containers fill by capillary action, the collection tip can be lightly touched to the drop of blood and the blood will be drawn into the container. Collection devices should not touch the puncture site and should not be scraped over the skin, because this will produce specimen contamination and hemolysis. Fingers are positioned slightly downward but with the palmar surface facing down during the collection procedure (Figure 6–9).

To prevent introduction of air bubbles, capillary tubes and micropipets are held horizontally while being filled. The presence of air bubbles limits the amount of blood that can be collected per tube and interferes with blood gas determinations and tests performed with Unopettes. When the tubes are filled, they are sealed with sealant clay or designated plastic caps.

Figure 6-9

Specimen collection from the finger

(From Strasinger, SK, and Di Lorenzo, MA: Phlebotomy Workbook for the Multiskilled Healthcare Professional. FA Davis, Philadelphia, 1996, Figure 16–8, p. 271, with permission.)

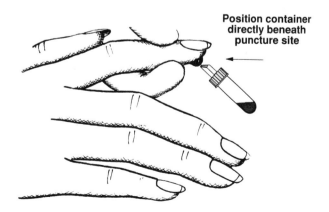

Position container directly beneath puncture site

While collecting the sample, the patient's hand does not have to be completely turned over. Rotating the hand 90 degrees allows blood collectors to clearly see the blood drops without placing themselves in awkward positions.

Microcollection tubes are slanted down during the collection, and blood is allowed to run through the capillary collection scoop and down the side of the tube. The tip of the collection container is placed beneath the puncture site and touches the underside of the drop. The first 3 drops of blood provide the channel to allow blood to flow freely into the container. Gently tapping the bottom of the tube may be necessary to force blood to the bottom. When a tube is filled, the color-coded top is attached. Tubes with anticoagulants should be inverted 8 to 10 times. If blood flow is slow, it may be necessary to mix the tube while the collection is in progress. It is important to work quickly, because blood that takes more than 2 minutes to collect may form microclots in an anticoagulated microtainer.

When sufficient blood has been collected, pressure is applied to the puncture site with sterile gauze. The finger or heel is elevated and pressure is applied until the bleeding stops. Make sure bleeding has stopped prior to removing the pressure.

Bandages are not used for children younger than 2 years of age because they may remove the bandages, place them in their mouth, and possibly aspirate the bandage. The adhesive may also cause irritation to sensitive skin.

Order of Collection

The order of draw for collecting multiple specimens from a dermal puncture is important because of the tendency of platelets to accumulate at the site of a wound. Blood to be used for tests for the evaluation of platelets, such as blood smear, platelet count, and CBC, must be collected first. The blood smear should be made first, followed by specimens for the Unopette platelet system or the lavender top Microtainer, other anticoagulated tubes, and then the clotted specimens.

LABELING THE SPECIMEN

Microsamples must be labeled with the same information required for venipuncture specimens. Labels can be wrapped around microcollection tubes or groups of capillary pipets. For transport, capillary pipets are then placed in a large tube, because the outside of the capillary pipets may be contaminated with blood. This procedure also helps prevent breakage.

Becton Dickinson Microtainer collection tubes have extenders that can be attached to the container. This allows the computer label to be applied vertically.

COMPLETION OF THE PROCEDURE

The dermal puncture procedure is completed by disposing of all used materials in appropriate containers, removing gloves, washing hands, and thanking the patient and/or the parents for their cooperation.

All special handling procedures associated with venipuncture specimens also apply to microspecimens.

To prevent excessive removal of blood from small infants, many nurseries have a log sheet for documenting the amount of blood collected each time a procedure is requested.

As with venipuncture, it is recommended that only two punctures be attempted to collect the blood. When a second puncture must be made to collect the sufficient amount of blood, the blood should not be added to the previously collected tube. This can cause erroneous results due to microclots and hemolysis.

SUMMARY OF THE DERMAL PUNCTURE PROCEDURE

1. Obtain and examine the requisition form.
2. Assemble equipment and supplies.
3. Greet the patient and/or the parents.
4. Identify the patient.
5. Position the patient and the parents.
6. Wash hands and put on gloves.
7. Organize equipment and supplies.
8. Select the puncture site.
9. Warm the puncture site if necessary.
10. Cleanse and allow the puncture site to dry.
11. Perform the puncture.
12. Wipe away the first drop of blood.
13. Make blood smears if requested.
14. Collect the hematology specimen and then other specimens.
15. Mix the specimens if necessary.
16. Apply pressure.
17. Dispose of the puncture device.
18. Label the specimens.
19. Perform appropriate specimen handling.
20. Examine the site for stoppage of bleeding.
21. Thank the patient and/or the parents.
22. Dispose of used supplies.
23. Remove and dispose of gloves.
24. Wash hands.
25. Complete any required paperwork.
26. Deliver specimens to the appropriate locations.

Evaluation of a Fingerstick

Rating System   **2 = Satisfactory**   **1 = Needs Improvement**   **0 = Incorrect/Did Not Perform**

_____ 1. Greets patient and explains procedure.
_____ 2. Examines requisition form.
_____ 3. Asks patient to state full name.
_____ 4. Compares requisition information and patient's statement.
_____ 5. Washes hands and puts on gloves.
_____ 6. Organizes and assembles equipment.
_____ 7. Selects appropriate finger.

_____ 8. Warms finger if necessary.
_____ 9. Gently massages finger.
_____ 10. Cleanses site with alcohol and allows it to air dry.
_____ 11. Does not contaminate puncture device.
_____ 12. Smoothly performs puncture across fingerprint.
_____ 13. Wipes away first drop of blood.

_____ 14. Collects two microhematocrit tubes without air bubbles.

_____ 15. Seals tubes.

_____ 16. Cleanses site and asks patient to apply pressure.

_____ 17. Labels tubes.

_____ 18. Examines site for stoppage of bleeding and applies bandage.

_____ 19. Thanks patient.

_____ 20. Disposes of puncture device in sharps container.

_____ 21. Disposes of used supplies.

_____ 22. Removes gloves.

_____ 23. Washes hands.

Total points _____
Maximum points = 46
COMMENTS

UNIT 1 INTRODUCTION TO PHLEBOTOMY

Introduction
    Course Purpose
    Course Overview
Importance of Correct Specimen Collection and Handling
    Specimen Integrity
    Influencing Factors
Safety Precautions
    Standard Precautions
    Risks Associated with Blood Collection
        Significant Exposure
        Syringe to Tube Blood Transfer
        Specimen Processing
    Needle Disposal
Types of Specimens
    Whole blood
    Plasma
    Serum
    Anticoagulant Mechanism
    Hemolyzed Specimens
    Icteric Specimens
    Lipemic Specimens
    Arterial Blood Specimens
    Capillary Blood Specimens
Quality Assurance

UNIT 2 VENIPUNCTURE EQUIPMENT

Introduction
Organization of Equipment
    Phlebotomy Trays
    Drawing Stations
Evacuated Tube System
    Needles
        Gauges
        Structure
        Safety Needles
    Adapters/Holders
        Purpose
        Assembly

Needle Disposal Systems
    Puncture-resistant Containers
    Retractable Needles
    Automatic Needle Removal
    Manual Needle Removal
    Safety Methods
Collection Tubes
    Description
    Rubber Stoppers
    Hemogard Closures
    Color-coding
        Lavender
            Anticoagulant
            Purpose
            Tests
        Light-blue
            Anticoagulant
            Purpose
            Tests
            Blood:Liquid Ratio
            Soybean Trypsin Inhibitor
        Black
            Anticoagulant
            Purpose
            Test
        Green
            Anticoagulant
            Purpose
            Tests
        Light-green/Green/Black
            Plasma Separator Tube (PST)
            Tests
        Yellow/Gray (Orange Hemogard)
            Additive
            Purpose
            Tests
        Gray
            Additives
            Purpose
            Tests

Royal Blue
  Characteristics
  Stoppers
  Additives
  Tests
Brown
  Characteristics
  Test
Yellow
  Two Types
  Additives
  Purpose
  Tests
Red/Gray (Gold Hemogard)
  Serum Separator Tube (SST)
  Additives
  Principles
  Tests
Red
  Purpose
  Tests
Order of Draw
  Principle
  Examples
  Evacuated Tube Order
Syringes
  Description/Uses
  Protective Sheath/Shields
  Transfer of Blood to Evacuated Tubes
  Order of Tube Transfer
Winged Infusion Sets
  Description/Uses
  Protective Safety Devices
  Uses
Tourniquets
  Types
  Purpose
Gloves
Antiseptics
  Isopropyl Alcohol
  Iodine/Chlorhexidine
Gauze/Bandages
Additional Supplies
  Pens
  Biohazard Transport Bags
Quality Control
  Sterility
  Visual Inspection
  Evacuated Tubes
    Lot Numbers
    Expiration Dates
  Possible Errors

UNIT 3 ROUTINE VENIPUNCTURE

Blood Collection Procedure
  Requisitions
    Purpose

Formats
  Information Required
Greeting the Patient
Patient Identification
  Importance
  Requisition Verification
  Verbal
  Identification Band Information
  Blood Bank Identification Systems
  Unidentified Patients
Patient Preparation
  Patient Reassurance
  Verify Patient's Pretest Conditions (Fasting, etc.)
  Variables
  Positioning the Patient
Handwashing and Gloving
Equipment Selection
Tourniquet Application
  Function
  Length of Application
  Tests Affected by Prolonged Application
  Location
  Technique
Site Selection
  Major Veins
  Palpation
    Technique
    Differentiation Between Tendons and Arteries
  Techniques to Enhance Vein Prominence
  Alternate Sites
    Hands
    Legs
  Sites to Avoid
    Occluded Veins
    Hematomas
    Edematous Areas
    Burns and Scars
    Mastectomies
    IVs
    Fistulas
Cleansing the Site
  Antiseptics
  Technique
  Drying
  Blood Alcohol Collection
Examination of Puncture Equipment
  Needle Defects
  Defective Evacuated Tubes
Performing the Venipuncture
  Holding the Needle Assembly
  Anchoring the Vein
  Puncture Angle
  Advancing and Changing Tubes
  Mixing
  Removing Needle
  Applying Pressure
Disposal of Needle

Labeling the Tubes
  Methods
    Required Information
  Inspection of the Site
  Bandaging
    Methods
    Excessive Bleeding
  Disposal of Used Supplies
  Thanking the Patient
  Laboratory Specimen Delivery
    Timing
    Processing

UNIT 4 COMPLICATIONS AND ADDITIONAL TECHNIQUES

Failure to Obtain Blood
  Adjusting Needle in Veins
  Collapsed Veins
  Probing
  Number of Resticks
Hematomas
  Failure to Remove Tourniquets
  Inadequate Pressure
  Probing
  Needle Not in Vein
  Needle Going Through Vein
  Bending the Elbow for Pressure
Hemolysis
  Tests Affected
  Causes
    Small-Gauge Needle
    Small-Gauge Needle and Large Tube
    Loose Syringe Needle
    Rapidly Pulling Back Syringe Plunger
    Drawing from a Hematoma
    Vigorous Mixing
    Forcing Blood from a Syringe into a Tube
Specimen Contamination
  Edema
  Hematomas
  IVs
  Alcohol
  Anticoagulant Carryover
Other Technical Problems
  Maintaining Pressure on Evacuated Tubes
  Reflux
  Partially Filled Collection Tubes
Patient Complications
  Syncope
  Seizure
  Petechiae
  Preanalytical Variables
Syringes
  Advantages
  Technique
  Disposal
  Transferring Blood from a Syringe to a Tube
Winged Infusion Sets
  Advantages

  Technique
  Disposal
Central Venous Catheters
  Special Requirements
  Types
  Discard Volumes
  Order of Collection
Specimen Rejection
  Unlabeled and Mislabeled
  Inadequate Volume
  Wrong Tube
  Hemolysis
  Lipemia
  Clotted Anticoagulated Specimen
  Improper Special Handling
  No Requisition Form
  Contaminated Containers

UNIT 5 SPECIAL VENIPUNCTURE COLLECTION

Fasting and Timed Specimens
  Two-Hour Postprandial Glucose
  Glucose Tolerance Test (GTT)
    Fasting Specimens
    Glucose Administration
    Specimen Timing
    Specimen Labeling
    Venipuncture versus Dermal Puncture
    Vomiting
  Diurnal Variation
  Therapeutic Drug Monitoring
    Trough Levels
    Peak Levels
    Specimen Labeling
Blood Cultures
  Timing
    Routine Sets
    Temperature Spikes
    Preantibiotic Administration
  Procedure
    Collection from Multiple Sites
    Equipment
    Aseptic Collection and Transfer
    Anticoagulant
    Site Preparation
    Aerobic and Anaerobic Specimens
    Ratio of Blood to Culture Media
Special Specimen Handling Procedures
  Cold Agglutinins
  Chilled Specimens
  Specimens Sensitive to Light
  Legal Specimens
    Chain of Custody
    Legal Blood Alcohol Collection

UNIT 6 DERMAL PUNCTURE

Introduction
    Increased Performance of Dermal Punctures
    Infants and Children

Complications of Deep Vein Punctures
    Cardiac Arrest
    Venous Thrombosis
    Hemorrhage
    Tissue and Organ Damage
    Infection
    Arteriospasm
    Restraining Injuries
Adults
    Burns and Scars
    Chemotherapy Patients
    Thrombotic Tendencies
    Geriatric Patients
    Inaccessible Veins
    Glucose Monitoring
Importance of Correct Collection
    Composition of Capillary Blood
    Volume of Blood Hemolysis
    Arterial versus Venous Blood
    Difference in Chemical Concentrations
Dermal Puncture Equipment
    General Equipment
    Skin Puncture Devices
        Puncture Depth
        Puncture Width
        Manual and Automatic Devices
    Microspecimen Containers
        Capillary Tubes
        Micropipets
        Microcollection Tubes
        Micropipet and Dilution System
Dermal Puncture Procedure
    Prepuncture Preparation
        Requisition and Equipment Selection
        Patient Identification
        Notation of Dermal Puncture on Requisition Form
    Patient Preparation
        Site Warming
    Site Selection
        Precautions
        Areas to Avoid

        Callused
        Bruised
        Scarred
        Edematous
        Infected
        Previous Punctures
    Heel Puncture Sites
        Plantar Surface
        Avoiding the Calcaneus and Arch
    Finger Puncture Sites
        Age and Tissue Restrictions
        Palmar Sites
        Fingers of Choice
Cleansing the Site
    Procedure
    Interference from Alcohol
        Stinging Sensation
        Specimen Contamination
        Hemolysis
        Inability to Obtain a Rounded Drop
Performing the Puncture
    Holding the Heel or Finger
    Massaging
    Direction of Puncture
Specimen Collection
    Wiping Away the First Drop
    Excessive Milking versus Pressure
    Positioning of the Collection Container
    Order of Collection
    Completion of the Procedure
        Pressure
        Bandages
Labeling the Specimen
    Information
    Methods
Completion of the Procedure
    Disposing of Supplies
    Specimen Handling
    Completion of Log Sheets
Failure to Obtain Enough Blood

1. The safest, most economical method for performing routine venipunctures is use of:
   - **A.** Winged infusion sets
   - **B.** Plastic syringes
   - **C.** Glass syringes
   - **D.** Evacuated tubes

2. Which of the following tubes contains an anticoagulant that does not bind calcium?
   - **A.** Light-blue
   - **B.** Green
   - **C.** Gray
   - **D.** Lavender

3. An incompletely filled light-blue stopper tube should be:
   - **A.** Used only for prothrombin times
   - **B.** Checked for clots
   - **C.** Used only for glucose testing
   - **D.** Discarded

4. Use of a 23-gauge needle and a 15-mL evacuated tube may:
   - **A.** Produce an incompletely filled tube
   - **B.** Cause a clotted lavender top tube
   - **C.** Cause hemolysis
   - **D.** Produce a loss of vacuum

5. Using an evacuated tube system, the order of draw for a PTT, CBC, glucose, and crossmatch is:
   - **A.** Light-blue, lavender, gray, red
   - **B.** Red, lavender, light-blue, gray
   - **C.** Red, light-blue, lavender, gray
   - **D.** Lavender, red, light-blue, gray

6. Contamination of a red stopper tube with the anticoagulant from a lavender top tube will cause a falsely:
   - **A.** Decreased calcium value
   - **B.** Decreased glucose value
   - **C.** Increased glucose value
   - **D.** Increased calcium value

7. Correct patient identification should include matching all of the following EXCEPT:
   - **A.** Requisition forms
   - **B.** Bed signs
   - **C.** Wrist ID bands
   - **D.** Patients verbally stating their names

8. Correct palpation of a vein includes all of the following EXCEPT:
   A. Determining the depth of the vein
   B. Detecting a pulse using the thumb
   C. Determining the direction of the vein
   D. Probing with the index finger

9. The veins that are the easiest to anchor are the:
   A. Hand veins
   B. Cephalic veins
   C. Basilic veins
   D. Median cubital veins

10. Bracing the hand holding the needle assembly against the patient's arm:
    A. Decreases patient discomfort
    B. Prevents excess needle movement
    C. Decreases the possibility of hemolysis
    D. Causes the tubes to fill more quickly

11. When performing a venipuncture, the vein is anchored to:
    A. Prevent patient discomfort
    B. Increase its visibility
    C. Prevent rolling
    D. Allow use of a smaller needle

12. When performing a venipuncture, the needle is positioned at a:
    A. 40-degree angle with the bevel up
    B. 20-degree angle with the bevel down
    C. 15-degree angle with the bevel up
    D. 35-degree angle with the bevel down

13. After applying the tourniquet, blood should be drawn within:
    A. 30 seconds
    B. 1 minute
    C. 5 minutes
    D. 10 minutes

14. When pressure is applied to the puncture site, the:
    A. Patient's elbow should be bent
    B. Patient should be lying down
    C. Patient's arm should be straight
    D. Blood collector should use a pressure bandage

15. Collection tubes should be labeled:
    A. After returning to the laboratory
    B. Before leaving the patient
    C. Before collecting the specimen
    D. Prior to mixing

16. An example of improper disposal of venipuncture supplies and equipment is:
    A. Placing gauze and alcohol pads in a biohazard container
    B. Recapping the needle
    C. Removing gloves and washing hands
    D. Placing the plastic needle cover in the wastebasket

17. When collecting blood from a patient with an IV in the right arm and a large hematoma in the antecubital area of the left arm, the blood collector should collect the specimen from:
    A. Below the hematoma
    B. Above the hematoma
    C. The antecubital area of the right arm
    D. The antecubital area of the left arm

18. When specimens are collected from an indwelling line:
    A. Lines do not need to be flushed following collection
    B. Coagulation tests are collected first
    C. The first 5 mL of blood must be discarded
    D. The tubes do not need to be mixed

19. When collecting blood using a butterfly, all of the following are acceptable EXCEPT:
    A. Lowering the angle of insertion
    B. Drawing blood into a syringe
    C. Using a 15-mL evacuated tube
    D. Threading the needle into the vein

20. When blood is collected from an intravenous line:
    A. This should be noted on the requisition form
    B. The physician should be notified
    C. The IV fluid should not be restarted
    D. A butterfly apparatus should be used

21. Hematomas can be caused by all of the following EXCEPT:
    A. Having the patient bend the elbow
    B. Inserting the needle partially into the vein
    C. Drawing below an IV line
    D. Removing the tourniquet after removing the needle

22. The number and size of syringes needed to collect a blood culture and a prothrombin time from a CVC is:
    A. Two 5-mL and one 10-mL   C. One 5-mL and two 10-mL
    B. One 5-mL and one 20-mL   D. Two 5-mL and one 30-mL

23. Forcing blood from a syringe into an evacuated tube may:
    A. Increase potassium values   C. Produce lipemic serum
    B. Decrease glucose values   D. Contaminate a blood culture

24. All of the following specimens would be rejected EXCEPT a(an):
    A. Unlabeled specimen
    B. Half-full red stopper tube
    C. Half-full light-blue stopper tube
    D. Specimen without a requisition form

25. The timing for a GTT begins:
    A. After collection of the fasting sample
    B. When the patient begins drinking the glucose
    C. When the patient finishes drinking the glucose
    D. 30 minutes after the glucose is finished

26. The order in which cleansing solutions are applied to the patient's arm before and after the collection of a blood culture is:
    A. Soap, alcohol, iodine   C. Iodine, alcohol, soap
    B. Alcohol, iodine, alcohol   D. Alcohol, alcohol, iodine

27. Three blood cultures from a patient requiring ASAP administration of antibiotics are collected:
    A. Every 30 minutes
    B. Before, during, and after the antibiotic is administered
    C. Immediately from three different sites
    D. Before, during, and after the fever spikes

28. An acceptable method for transporting a specimen that requires chilling is:
   A. Submersion in cold water
   B. Submersion in crushed ice
   C. Chilling the tube prior to collection
   D. In a plastic bag containing ice cubes

29. Use of evacuated tubes after their expiration date may result in:
   A. No clot formation in red top tubes
   B. Consistently elevated results
   C. Consistently decreased results
   D. Clot formation in lavender stopper tubes

30. Using a lancet that produces a puncture deeper than recommended may cause:
   A. Septicemia
   B. Hemolysis
   C. Osteomyelitis
   D. Specimen contamination

31. All of the following are acceptable skin puncture devices EXCEPT:
   A. Lancets
   B. Surgical blades
   C. Autolets
   D. Tenderfoots

32. Failure to puncture across the fingerprint during a finger puncture will cause:
   A. Blood to run down the finger
   B. Hemolysis
   C. Contamination of the specimen
   D. Additional patient discomfort

33. A blood collector is recollecting a dermal puncture specimen because of hemolysis. The patient complains about a stinging sensation from the first puncture. The most probable cause of the hemolysis in the first specimen is:
   A. Not allowing alcohol to dry
   B. Excessive massaging
   C. Vigorous mixing of the microtube
   D. Use of a small lancet

Laboratory Tests and the Required Types of Anticoagulants and Volume of Blood Required

Test	Collection Tube	Minimum Amount	Comments
Ammonia	Dark-green	3 mL	Send on ice
Amylase	Light-green PST/Gold SST	3 mL	
Antibiotic assay (Gent, Tob, Vanco)	Red clot/clear nongel Microtainer	5 mL /(0.5 mL)	No SST tubes
Antibody ID/Screen	Lavender	7 mL	Blood bank ID
Beta HCG/Quant.	Light-green PST/Gold SST	3 mL	
Bilirubin	Gold SST/Amber Microtainer	1.5 mL /(0.5 mL)	Protect from light
B_{12}	Gold SST/Red clot	3 mL	
CBC	Lavender	3 mL	
Cortisol	Gold SST/Red clot	2 mL	Serum only
Cross-match	Lavender	7 mL	Blood bank ID remains on 72 hours
D-Dimer	Light-blue	4.5 mL	Tube must be full (stable for 4 hours)
Ethanol/Alcohol	Red clot/Gray	3 mL	Do not open tube until testing
Fibrinogen	Light-blue	4.5 mL	Tube must be full
Folate	Gold SST/Red clot	3 mL	
Glucose	Light-green/Gold SST	3 mL	
Hgb/Hct	Lavender	3 mL	
Hepatitis panels	Gold SST/Red clot	6 mL	
Ionized calcium	Gold SST/Red clot/Arterial gas syringe	7 mL	Tube must be full; may use arterial gas syringe
Lactate	Green/arterial gas syringe	5 mL	Send in ice; analyze in 15 minutes
Lead	Royal blue EDTA	6 mL	
Lipase	Light-green PST/Gold SST	3 mL	
Lithium	Gold SST/Red clot	5 mL	Draw 12 hours post dose
MI panel (myo, CK-MB, troponin)	Light-green PST	3 mL	Stable 4 hours
Monospot	Gold SST/Red clot	3 mL	
PH	Dark-green on ice	3 mL	Send on ice
Platelet	Lavender	3 mL	
Prothrombin time (PT)	Light-blue	4.5 mL	Full tube; stable 4 hours refrigerated
PTT/APTT	Light-blue	4.5 mL	Full tube; stable 4 hours refrigerated

(Continued)

Test	Collection Tube	Minimum Amount	Comments
Protein electrophoresis	Gold SST/Red clot	3 mL	
Reticulocyte count	Lavender	3 mL	
Therapeutic drugs (digoxin, Theo, Pheno, Pheny, Carb, Val Ac.)	Red clot/Clear nongel Microtainer	3 mL/(full Microtainer)	No SST tubes
TSH/Free T4	Light-green/Gold SST	3 mL	
Quant proteins (C3, C4, IgG, IgA, IgM, haptoglobin)	Gold SST/Red clot	3 mL	
Sedimentation rate (ESR)	Lavender	5 mL	
Chemistry panels (renal, hepatic, comprehensive, metabolic)	Light-green/Gold SST	3 mL	
Lipid panel (HDL, Chol, Trig)	Gold SST	5 mL	

APTT, activated partial thromboplastin time; Carb, carbamazepine; CBC, complete blood count; Chol, cholesterol; CK-MB, isoenzyme of creatine kinase with muscle and brain subunits; ESR, erythrocyte sedimentation rate; Gent, gentamicin; HCG, human chorionic gonadotropin; Hct, hematocrit; HDL, high-density lipoprotein; Hgb, hemoglobin; ID, identification; Ig, immunoglobin; MI, myocardial infarction; myo, myoglobin; pH, hydrogen ion concentration; Pheno, phenobarbital; Pheny, phenytoin; PST, plasma separator tube; PTT, partial thromboplastin time; Quant., quantitative; SST, serum separator tube; T4, thyroxine; Theo, theophylline; Tob, tobramycin; Trig, triglycerides; TSH, thyroid-stimulating hormone; Val ac., valproic acid; Vanco, Vancomycin.

This is a list of anticoagulant and specimen requirements for the most common test requests at Methodist Hospital, Omaha, Nebraska, courtesy of Diane Wolff, MT(ASCP), Phlebotomy Supervisor. Each laboratory will have specific test protocols.

APPENDIX 4

IV Access:
Flush Protocols

	Peripheral	Central Venous Catheter	Hickman	Groshong	Implanted Ports (Open or Closed)	Quenton/ Sheldon Catheter	Arterial Lines Radial/ Femoral	PICC Lines	CATH LINK	Midline Catheter
		Subclavian or jugular (single, double, or triple) Triple lumen use: • Distal for meds, TPN • Medial for blood infusion • Proximal for lab draws	Single, double; each lumen capped with needleless cap	Single or double lumen; each lumen capped with needleless cap	Single or double port, open or closed-ended	Dialysis only unless physician order for IV use; double lumen		Peripherally Inserted Central Catheter (open or closed-ended)	Implanted vascular port	
Access	If converted to saline lock, must have additional tubing.	Each port capped with needleless cap.			Access through skin using right-angle noncoring needle. **Do not** aspirate for placement, as flush will indicate placement.		Pressure tubing to arterial catheter	Through one vein of antecubital fossa and tip ending in superior vena cava	Use an IV 20-gauge, 2-inch catheter. **Never use noncoring needle.**	Through one vein of antecubital fossa with tip ending in upper arm, below axillary vein
IV ports prepping	Alcohol	Alcohol wipe	Alcohol wipe	Alcohol wipe	Betadine application for skin prep; alcohol prep for prepping IV ports	Alcohol wipe	Remove sterile cap prior to access	Alcohol wipe	Alcohol wipe	Alcohol wipe
IV tubing changes	Every 72 hours	Every 72 hours	Every 72 hours	Every 72 hours	Every 72 hours	Every 72 hours or with dialysis	Every 72 hours	Every 72 hours	Every 72 hours	Every 72 hours
TPN tubing changes	Every 24 hours	Every 24 hours	Every 24 hours	Every 24 hours	Every 24 hours	Every 24 hours		Every 24 hours	Every 24 hours	Every 24 hours

	Peripheral	Central Venous Catheter	Hickman	Groshong	Implanted Ports (Open or Closed)	Quenton/ Sheldon Catheter	Arterial Lines Radial/ Femoral	PICC Lines	CATH LINK	Midline Catheter
Secondary tubing changes	If used continuously, change 72 hours. If not in use within 24 hours, discard.	If used continuously, change 72 hours. If not in use within 24 hours, discard.	If used continuously, change 72 hours. If not in use within 24 hours, discard.	If used continuously, change 72 hours. If not in use within 24 hours, discard.	If used continuously, change 72 hours. If not in use within 24 hours, discard.	If used continuously, change 72 hours. If not in use within 24 hours, discard.	If used continuously, change 72 hours. If not in use within 24 hours, discard.	If used continuously, change 72 hours. If not in use within 24 hours, discard.	If used continuously, change 72 hours. If not in use within 24 hours, discard.	If used continuously, change 72 hours. If not in use within 24 hours, discard.
Fat filter	24 hours	24 hours	24 hours	24 hours	24 hours	24 hours		24 hours	24 hours	24 hours
Between med infusion	2 mL N.S.	2 mL N.S. followed by 1.5 mL heparinized saline	5 mL N.S. followed by 1.5 mL heparinized saline	5 mL N.S.	5 mL N.S.			*Closed: Meds:* 5 cc N.S. before med, 20 cc N.S. after *TPN:* 10 mL N.S. before med, 20 mL saline *Open: Meds:* 5 mL saline before med; 20 mL N.S. after med, followed by 5 mL) heparinized saline (100 U/1 mL) *TPN:* 10 mL saline before, 20 mL saline after TPN, followed by 5 mL heparinized saline (100 U/1 mL)	10 cc N.S. before med. 10 mL N.S. after med/ TPN followed by 5 mL (100 U/1 mL) heparinized saline	Meds: 5 cc N.S. before med, 5 cc N.S. after med *TPN:* 10 cc N.S. before med, 10 cc N.S. after med

	Peripheral	Central Venous Catheter	Hickman	Groshong	Implanted Ports Open or Closed	Quenton/ Sheldon Catheter	Arterial Lines Radial/ Femoral	PICC Lines	CATH LINK	Midline Catheter
Not in use	2 mL N.S. every 12 hours	Every 12 hours 2 mL N.S. followed by 1.5 mL heparinized saline (each lumen)	5 mL N.S., 1.5 mL heparinized saline weekly	5 mL N.S. weekly	5 mL N.S. monthly; if open: follow with 5 mL heparinized (100 U/1 mL) to port			Closed: 5 mL N.S. weekly Open: 5 mL heparinized saline (100 U/1 mL) every day	If catheter not in place: every 30 days 10 cc N.S. followed by 5 mL (100 U/1 mL) heparinized saline. If catheter in place, but not using: flush every 8 hours with 10 mL N.S. followed by 5 mL (100 U/1 mL) heparinized saline.	5 cc weekly and PRN
Dressing changes	When IV site is changed or every 72 hours, or if integrity of dressing is compromised	Day after insertion, then 72 hours, or if integrity of dressing is compromised	Day after insertion, then 72 hours, or if integrity of dressing is compromised	Day after insertion, then 72 hours, or if integrity of dressing is compromised	Weekly and PRN	Every 72 hours or with dialysis	Day after insertion and then every 72 hours or if integrity of dressing compromised	Day after insertion and then every 72 hours or if integrity of dressing compromised	72 hours	Day after insertion, weekly and PRN
Cap/needle changes	With site change or with each LAV use; site changed every 72 hours	Weekly and PRN	Weekly and PRN	Weekly or whenever cap is removed	Weekly for needles	Change cap with every dialysis or weekly	Change dead end cap with each blood draw	Weekly or whenever cap is removed	Change needle weekly	Weekly or whenever cap is removed

	Peripheral	Central Venous Catheter	Hickman	Groshong	Implanted Ports Open or Closed	Quenton/ Sheldon Catheter	Arterial Lines Radial/ Femoral	PICC Lines	CATH LINK	Midline Catheter
Flush, how often	Every 12 hours and after each use	Every 12 hours and after every use	Weekly and after each use, or if cap has been removed, cap appears damaged or is leaking, or blood in cap	Weekly and after each use, or if cap has been removed, cap appears damaged or is leaking, or blood in cap	Monthly and after each use	After each use	Continuous heparinized flush	*Closed:* every week and after each use. *Open:* daily or after every use.	After each use. If not in use, weekly, if catheter in place. If no catheter, every 4 weeks.	After each use, weekly and PRN
Flush solutions and volume	2 mL N.S. (not heparinized)	2 mL N.S. followed by 1.5 mL heparinized saline (each lumen)	5 mL N.S. followed by 1.5 mL heparinized saline (each lumen)	5 mL N.S. not heparinized (use 10 mL saline if blood observed in cath) (each lumen)	5 mL N.S. *Open:* follow with 5 mL heparinized saline (100 U/1 mL) to port	10 mL N.S. followed with 0.4 cc of 10,000 U/cc of heparin and 0.9 cc N.S. to equal 1.3 cc of solution to each lumen	N.S. 500 mL with 1000 U heparin using pressure bag inflated to 300 mg Hg	*Closed:* 5 cc N.S. *Open:* 5 cc N.S. followed by 5 cc heparin (100 U/1 mL) every day	10 cc N.S. followed by 5 mL (100 U/1 mL) heparinized saline	5 cc sterile saline

(Continued)

Arterial Lines

	Peripheral	Central Venous Catheter	Hickman	Groshong	Implanted Ports	PICC	Radial Arterial Lines	Femoral Line	CATH LINK	Midline Catheter
Blood Draw	Flush each lumen	5 mL N.S. if IV solution will interfere with lab studies	5 mL N.S. if IV solution will interfere with lab studies	10 mL N.S. if TPN or blood and if blood coagulation studies ordered; flush with 20 mL N.S.	5 mL N.S. if IV solution will interfere with lab studies	10 mL N.S. if TPN, flush with 20 mL N.S.	Turn stopcock off to pressure bag. **Do not use** line for blood cultures.	Turn stopcock off to pressure bag.	Implanted port 10 mL N.S. if IV solution will interfere with lab studies.	Flush each lumen: 10 cc N.S. If TPN infusing, flush with 20 cc N.S.
With IV Infusing — Clamp each lumen/tubing prior to draw	1 minute	1 minute	1 minute	Do not clamp—stop all IVs infusing	1 minute	1 minute			1 minute	Clamp each lumen; wait 1 minute
Discard	2 mL	3 mL	6 mL	6 mL	3 mL	3 mL	5 mL with syringe	10 mL with syringe	6 mL	3 mL
Withdraw blood sample	Based on test	Based on test	Based on test	Based on test	Based on test	Based on test	According to lab specimen	According to lab specimen	Based on test	Based on test
Flush each lumen after draw	2 mL, resume infusion	5 mL N.S., resume infusion all lumens	10 mL, resume infusion	10 mL, resume infusion	10 mL, resume infusion	20 mL N.S., resume infusion	Turn stopcock toward patient; flush stopcock using sterile syringe; replace with new sterile cap, then flush line via transducer, manually until line clear and verify wave form	Turn stopcock toward patient; flush stopcock using sterile syringe; replace with new sterile cap, then flush line via transducer, manually until line clear and verify ware form	20 mL N.S., resume infusion	10 cc N.S., resume infusion

	Peripheral	Central Venous Catheter	Hickman	Groshong	Implanted Ports	PICC	Arterial Lines		CATH LINK	Midline Catheter
							Radial Arterial Lines	Femoral Line		
Without IV infusing Flush each lumen	2 mL N.S.	5 mL N.S.	5 mL N.S.	10 mL N.S.	5 mL N.S.	10 mL N.S.			10 mL N.S.	10 cc N.S.
Discard Withdraw blood sample	2 mL Based on test	3 mL Based on test	6 mL Based on test	6 mL Based on test	3 mL Based on test	3 mL Based on test			5 mL Based on test	3 mL Based on test
Flush each lumen after draw	2 mL	5 mL N.S. followed with 1.5 mL heparinized saline (100 U/1 mL)	*Flush: 5 mL N.S. followed by 1.5 mL heparinized saline (100 U/1 mL)	Flush: 10 mL N.S.	If closed, flush 10 mL saline. If open ended, flush 10 mL saline followed with 5 mL heparinized saline (100 U/1 mL).	If closed, flush 20 mL N.S. If open ended, follow with heparinized saline 5 mL (100 U/1 mL).			Flush with 20 mL N.S. followed by heparinized saline 5 cc (100 U/1 mL)	10 cc N.S.

N.S., normal saline; PRN, as needed; TPN, total parenteral nutrition.

*Note: If patient is undergoing transplant, question use of normal saline for flushing instead of heparin as heparin interferes with immunological response.

Courtesy of Patty Janousek, BSN, CRNI, Methodist Hospital, Omaha, NE 68114.

Clinical Correlations of Blood Tests Related to Body Systems

Test	Clinical Correlation
CIRCULATORY SYSTEM	
Activated clotting time (ACT)	Heparin therapy
Activated partial thromboplastin time [APTT(PTT)]	Heparin therapy or coagulation disorders
Antibody (Ab) screen	Blood transfusion
Antistreptolysin O (ASO) titer	Rheumatic fever
Antithrombin III	Coagulation disorders
Aspartate aminotransferase [AST(SGOT)]	Cardiac muscle damage
Bilirubin	Hemolytic disorders
Bleeding time (BT)	Platelet function
Blood culture	Septicemia
Blood group and type	ABO group and Rh factor
C-reactive protein (CRP)	Inflammatory disorders
Cholesterol	Coronary artery disease
Complete blood count (CBC)	Anemia, infection, leukemia, or bleeding disorders
Creatine kinase [CK(CPK)]	Myocardial infarction
Creatine kinase isoenzymes (CK-MB)	Myocardial infarction
Direct anti–human globulin test (DAT) or direct Coombs	Anemia or hemolytic disease of the newborn
Erythrocyte sedimentation rate (ESR)	Inflammatory disorders
Fibrin degradation products (FDP)	Disseminated intravascular coagulation
Fibrinogen	Coagulation disorders
Folate	Anemia
Hematocrit (Hct)	Anemia
Hemoglobin (Hgb)	Anemia
Hemoglobin (Hgb) electrophoresis	Hemoglobin abnormalities
High-density lipoprotein (HDL)	Coronary risk
Iron	Anemia
Lactate dehydrogenase [LD(LDH)]	Myocardial infarction
Low-density lipoprotein (LDL)	Coronary risk
Myoglobin	Myocardial infarction
Platelet (Plt) count	Bleeding tendencies
Prothrombin time (PT)	Coumadin therapy and coagulation disorders

(Continued)

Test	Clinical Correlation
CIRCULATORY SYSTEM	
Reticulocyte (Retic) count	Bone marrow function
Sickle cell screening	Sickle cell anemia
Total iron binding capacity (TIBC)	Anemia
Triglycerides	Coronary artery disease
Troponin	Myocardial infarction
Type and cross-match (T & C)	Blood transfusion
Type and screen	Blood transfusion
White blood cell (WBC) count	Infections or leukemia
Vitamin B$_{12}$	Anemia
LYMPHATIC SYSTEM	
Anti-HIV	Human immunodeficiency virus
Antinuclear antibody (ANA)	Systemic lupus erythematosus/autoimmune disorders
Complete blood count (CBC)	Infectious mononucleosis
Complement levels	Immune system function/autoimmune disorders
Fluorescent antinuclear antibody (FANA)	Systemic lupus erythematosus/autoimmune disorders
Immunoglobulin (Ig) levels	Immune system function
Monospot	Infectious mononucleosis
p24 antigen	Human immunodeficiency virus
Protein electrophoresis	Multiple myeloma
T-cell count	Immune function/HIV monitoring
Viral load	HIV monitoring
Western blot	Human immunodeficiency virus
SKELETAL SYSTEM	
Alkaline phosphatase (ALP)	Bone disorders
Antinuclear antibody (ANA)	Systemic lupus erythematosus/collagen disorders
Calcium (Ca)	Bone disorders
Fluorescent antinuclear antibody (FANA)	Systemic lupus erythematosus/collagen disorders
Phosphorus (P)	Skeletal disorders
Rheumatoid arthritis (RA)	Rheumatoid arthritis
Uric acid	Gout
MUSCULAR SYSTEM	
Creatinine kinase [CK(CPK)]	Muscle damage
Creatinine kinase isoenzymes (CK-MM)	Muscle damage
Lactic acid	Muscle disorders
Magnesium (Mg)	Musculoskeletal disorders
Myoglobin	Muscle damage
Potassium (K)	Muscle function
NERVOUS SYSTEM	
Creatinine kinase isoenzymes (CK-BB)	Brain damage
Drug screening	Therapeutic drug monitoring or drug abuse
Lead	Neurological function
Lithium (Li)	Antidepressant drug monitoring

(Continued)

Test	Clinical Correlation
RESPIRATORY SYSTEM	
Arterial blood gases (ABGs)	Acid-base balance
Cold agglutinins	Atypical pneumonia
Complete blood count (CBC)	Pneumonia
Electrolytes (Lytes)	Acid-base balance
DIGESTIVE SYSTEM	
Alanine aminotransferase [ALT(SGPT)]	Liver disorders
Albumin	Malnutrition or liver disorders
Alcohol	Intoxication/liver function
Alkaline phosphatase (ALP)	Liver disorders
Ammonia	Severe liver disorders
Amylase	Pancreatitis
Anti–hepatitis B surface antigen	Immunity to hepatitis B
Anti–hepatitis C virus	Viral hepatitis
Aspartate aminotransferase [AST(SGOT)]	Liver disorders
Bilirubin	Liver disorders
Carcinoembryonic antigen (CEA)	Carcinoma detection and monitoring
Complete blood count (CBC)	Appendicitis, peritonitis, or other infection
Gamma-glutamyltransferase (GGT)	Early liver disorders
Gastrin	Gastric malignancy
Hepatitis B surface antigen (HBsAg)	Hepatitis B screening
Lactate dehydrogenase [LD(LDH)]	Liver disorders
Lipase	Pancreatitis
Total protein (TP)	Liver disorders
URINARY SYSTEM	
Albumin	Kidney disorders
Antistreptolysin O (ASO) titer	Acute glomerulonephritis
Blood urea nitrogen (BUN)	Kidney disorders
Creatinine	Kidney disorders
Creatinine clearance	Glomerular filtration
Electrolytes (Lytes)	Fluid and electrolyte balance
Osmolality	Fluid and electrolyte balance
Total protein (TP)	Kidney disorders
Uric acid	Kidney disorders
ENDOCRINE SYSTEM	
Adrenocorticotropic hormone (ACTH)	Adrenal and pituitary gland function
Calcium (Ca)	Parathyroid function
Cortisol	Adrenal cortex function
Glucose	Hypoglycemia or diabetes mellitus
Glucose tolerance test (GTT)	Hypoglycemia or diabetes mellitus
Growth hormone (GH)	Pituitary gland function
Insulin	Glucose metabolism and pancreatic function
Parathyroid hormone (PTH)	Parathyroid function
Phosphorus (P)	Endocrine disorders
Testosterone	Testicular function
Thyroid function (T3, T4, TSH) studies	Thyroid function

(Continued)

Test	Clinical Correlation
REPRODUCTIVE SYSTEM	
Estradiol, estriol, and estrogen	Ovarian or placental function
Fluorescent treponemal antibody–absorbed (FTA-ABS)	Syphilis
Human chorionic gonadotropin (Beta HCG)	Pregnancy
Prostate-specific antigen (PSA)	Prostatic cancer
Prostatic acid phosphatase (PAP)	Prostatic cancer
Rapid plasma reagin (RPR)	Syphilis
Rubella titer	Immunity to German measles
Toxoplasma antibody screening	Toxoplasma infection
Venereal Disease Research Laboratory (VDRL)	Syphilis

Answer

Keys

VENIPUNCTURE SITUATIONS EXERCISE

1. Attach temporary identification to the patient. Use a commercial blood bank identification system.

2. Request another blood collector to collect the PT.

3. a. 2
   b. X
   c. 1

4. 2.7 mL in the light-blue stopper tube
   2.0 mL in the lavender stopper tube
   2.3 mL in the red stopper tube

5. a. One 5-mL syringe for discarding the first 5 mL of blood
   One 10-mL syringe for the CBC and chemistry profile
   One 5-mL syringe for the prothrombin time
   b. The specimen was collected from an IV line and the type of fluid being administered

6. a. Collapsed vein
   b. Use smaller evacuated tubes
   Use a syringe

7. a. Blood is leaking out of the vein into the tissue.
   b. Remove the needle and apply pressure.
   c. Use a 23-gauge needle with a syringe or butterfly.

8. a. The specimen contained small clots.
   b. The blood collector was busy with the patient and did not mix the specimen.
   c. Yes. Use one hand to mix the specimen as soon as the patient's head was lowered.

9. Inadequate pressure is being applied to the site. These patients are often taking anticoagulants and require additional pressure.

10. a. The specimen was hemolyzed.
    b. Do not leave the tourniquet on for more than 1 minute.
    Use a smaller evacuated tube.
    Avoid mixing the sample.
    If the blood is collected in a syringe, immediately transfer it to the evacuated tube.

SPECIAL VENIPUNCTURE COLLECTION EXERCISE

1. Has the patient been fasting for 12 hours?

2. Yes, the patient may be bleeding internally and must be monitored.

3. Check to be sure the patient is fasting. Draw the fasting specimen. Instruct the patient to eat a full breakfast and return exactly 2 hours after completing breakfast. Draw the 2-hour specimen.

4. Notify the supervisor or physician about the vomiting. If the physician cannot be reached in time, collect the 3-hour specimen and note the vomiting on the requisition.

5. Cortisol levels should be drawn between 0800 and 1000. Collect the specimen before the patient goes to physical therapy.

6. No. The 0800 request would be the trough level, and the 1200 request could be the peak level.

7. Yes. The patient needs to be started on antibiotics.

8. a. Aseptic technique was not followed. One specimen was collected in the wrong tube.
   b. The anticoagulant in the lavender stopper tube killed the bacteria.

9. The ammonia level will be decreased because the specimen was not chilled immediately. The cold agglutinin will be decreased because it was not kept warm. The CBC will be unaffected.

10. a. 1. How do you know you collected blood from the right person?
      2. How did you disinfect the person's arm?
      3. How do you know the specimen you drew from this patient did not get mixed up with another specimen?
    b. 1. The blood collector explains the appropriate identification procedure and identifies a witness.
      2. The blood collector explains the use of cleansing agents other than alcohol.
      3. The blood collector explains the chain of custody procedure and produces it as documentation.

COMPREHENSIVE TEST

1. D	12. C	23. A
2. B	13. B	24. B
3. D	14. C	25. C
4. C	15. B	26. B
5. C	16. B	27. C
6. A	17. A	28. B
7. B	18. C	29. D
8. B	19. C	30. C
9. D	20. A	31. B
10. B	21. C	32. A
11. C	22. A	33. A

Index

Page numbers followed by f indicate figures; page numbers followed by t indicate tables.